Jean, Warrior Princess

Be Transformed As You Brave Cancer's Storm

Jeanie Winebarger

Copyright © 2021, Jeanie Winebarger

All rights reserved. No part of this publication may be reproduced or transmitted in any form or by any means, electronic or mechanical, including photocopying and recording, or by any information storage and retrieval system, except in the case of brief quotations for use in articles and reviews, without written permission from the author.

The views expressed in this book are the author's and do not necessarily reflect those of the publisher.

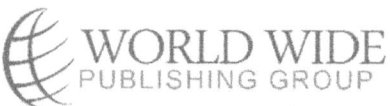

7710-T Cherry Park Dr, Ste 224
Houston, TX 77095
(713) 766-4271
Printed in the United States of America

Cover design by www.HarvestCreek.net

ISBN: 978-1-64830-252-7

Dedication

Dear Reader, I held you in my heart as I composed each line. This book is devoted to you. Your pilgrimage of healing, health, and faith will be followed by many. May my story give you the courage it takes to embrace life each moment, on the mountain top and in the valley. You are becoming the hero or heroine in your unique story as you actively embrace your new reality with resilience and laughter. You will come to know what it is to walk through the Valley of the Shadow and come out on the other side with greater strength and the determination of steel. Soon after my cancer diagnosis, there was one book I read over and over. Brett Farve's wife, Deanna Farve, wrote, *Don't Bet Against Me*. As I read, I walked with her from breast cancer diagnosis through treatment that included chemotherapy with all its side-effects, including low energy, nausea, and hair loss. I experienced her life, from the threat of defeat to health. Her crisis led to a more magnificent victory. I looked for other books like it - both personal and informative - but found none. I knew someone needed to hear my story too. I hope you will be comforted, obtain information, and receive support as you walk with me on my pathway of hope and healing.

Dear Family, I'm writing this for you. I want you to know what my life looks like, from the inside out. Be inspired to keep rising higher and stay the course, fearlessly moving through life's twists and turns.

I am writing for you, Dear Husband. We started this journey when we married in August 1970, not knowing what was in our future. All we knew was that we were madly in love, and we wanted to be together forever. We came together at the alter - two broken people who needed so much! Our two beautiful sons came along, God entered our lives, and we have made a wonderful life together. Through it all, we have learned to trust in our Father God and lean on His word more and more each day! You have released me to follow my dreams, including writing. I love you, Don! You make me laugh out loud every day. You have been my constant source of strength and love through it all!

Thank you, Dad, for naming me Jean, meaning the Lord is gracious. Though you transitioned from this present reality to the next life many years ago, I can still hear you call my name. When I was very young, that one-syllable name sounded hard and harsh to me. Now I understand that Jean was my fiercely serious name. Even then, you were growing me up to be brave. In my late teens, I wanted to soften the sound and asked everyone to call me Jeanie. Now, many years later, my heart jumps for joy when people call me Jean. Although God is full of mercy, truth, and grace, He is a warrior wanting to make things right. I want to be like my father God.

In this book, you will tour my crucible, day to day, week to week, month to month - from dreadful diagnosis to overcoming faith and new birth. A crucible is a situation or severe trial, in which different elements interact, leading to the creation of something new. You will experience the depths of raw emotions that come with life's most astonishing surprises. You will find new courage to conquer your fearful thoughts and situations. You will be empowered to trust God and yourself as you research and make wise decisions that may not always be conventional.

Contents

Foreword: Hope from the Heart of an Oncologist vii

Chapter 1: In The Beginning 1
Chapter 2: Moving Forward 7
Chapter 3: Managing Health and Wellness 11
Chapter 4: Being Brave 15
Chapter 5: Uncertain Testing Times 19
Chapter 6: Favorable Encounters And Choices 23
Chapter 7: Brave New World 27
Chapter 8: Medical Mystery Tour 31
Chapter 9: New Reality 35
Chapter 10: Facing The Giants 39
Chapter 11: Celebration Of Life 43
Chapter 12: Game Day 45
Chapter 13: Recovery Road 49
Chapter 14: Uncertainty 53
Chapter 15: Becoming The Warrior Princess 55
Chapter 16: Patient Persistence Through Threat and Pain 59
Chapter 17: Chemotherapy Champion 67

Chapter 18: Living Life on Different Levels 71
Chapter 19: Hair Today Gone Tomorrow 75
Chapter 20: Show Me Your Glory 81
Chapter 21: Little Lost Lamb 85
Chapter 22: Live Life Large In The Midst Of The Storm 89
Chapter 23: Chemo Change 93
Chapter 24: Perplexing Radiation Consultation 97
Chapter 25: From Suffering to Sharper Vision 103
Chapter 26: Mystery to Mastery 107
Chapter 27: Rocking, Reeling, and Working It Out 111
Chapter 28: Caregiver Perspective 115
Chapter 29: Question, Quest, Conquest 119
Chapter 30: Understanding Diverse and Complementary Options ... 125

Epilogue 131
The Poetic Warrior 131

Foreword

Hope from the Heart of an Oncologist

I get new breast cancer patients all the time, and I always encourage them. The world of cancer is quite diverse. Walking through the door, meeting a new patient is still a challenge. Some cancer diagnoses are more challenging to treat. I am not always as hopeful when treating some diseases, like pancreatic cancers or biliary cancers. Medical science has not put as much money into researching what causes them to develop and what drives them to be more aggressive. I'm not as optimistic about the outcome. However, when I get most breast cancer cases, I am more hopeful. We have made excellent progress with breast cancer research and patient support. We have so many different targeted therapies to choose from, including chemotherapy, molecular medicine, hormone therapy, and others. I don't want anybody to have cancer, but I would take a breast cancer case over many other cancer types anytime.

First, from an oncology standpoint, we have achieved a lot in the advancement of breast cancer diagnosis and treatment, and it's only getting better. That's encouraging. The second thing is that our society has embraced breast cancer for whatever reason and in a commendable way. The public does not give the same attention to colon, prostate, and other cancers, although they are also worthy of our investigation. Perhaps it's because our mothers, daughters, and wives get breast cancer. Football players wearing pink cleats in October, and there are fund-raising runs galore. People donate money all the time to breast cancer research. The information found through research brings a lot of support for the oncologist to develop new, more targeted medical options. Everyone wants to get behind breast cancer patients. Family and friends see you with the outward side-effects of treatment - hair loss and debilitation. They are on your side. You may be embarrassed by your bald head, but everyone else sees that as a badge of honor. The community wants to say, "Go get 'em! You can do it!"

And the last thing, I find women with breast cancer and cancer patients, in general, have a lot of faith. No, cancer is not fun. Yes, this is a bad thing happening to a good person. However, I have patients who see this as part of a mysterious plan for their life. People have not chosen this fearful event. A cancer diagnosis is not easy to understand or navigate. I don't want to use one of those cliches, but I think there is redemption in everything. I've seen some patients, who were inspired by their cancer journey, bring people to Christ. They are going through hell, but they are still praying, loving, and showing people who Christ is at a difficult time. They live out the verse in Philippians that says, *For me to live is Christ, and to die is gain.* From NIV. They are saying, 'I'm here, I'm living. I'm going to live out my faith. But if something happens, I will miss this beautiful world. I'll miss the sunsets. I'll miss my family. But the best day of my existence on earth does not compare to what it will be like when I enter the throne-room of heaven.' If my patient has a lot of faith or even a little bit, I ask them to take some time and use this moment in your life to build your trust in God. During this trial, you may be able to strengthen someone else's faith. Your husband is watching you. Your kids and your grandkids are watching you. Your redemption in this cancer may be that by showing God's love and grace, somebody else may want to experience His love and grace.

Jeanie Winebarger and her husband, Don, came to my office following her breast cancer diagnosis and subsequent bilateral mastectomy. They were both afraid yet hopeful. The diagnosis had disoriented them, and both were full of questions. Jeanie always arrived with her notebook and a list of items to discuss. She always took notes. When she posed a question that I could not answer off the top of my head, I researched the topic for her on the spot. She never left my office with an unanswered question. Her loving husband supported her all the way, and I never saw one without the other. At each visit, I complimented Jeanie on her blood work and her fancy head dressings. She took responsibility for doing her part, supporting chemotherapy treatment with a good diet. She also came to me full of faith while wading through the quicksand of her fear.

This book is a personal journal of one who walked with God, family, faith, and the best medical care. Read it and be encouraged.

--**Dr. Marc Usrey,** American Board of Internal Medicine- Medical Oncology, American Board of Internal Medicine-Hematology, UT Health East Texas, Hope Cancer Center, Tyler, Texas

Chapter 1

IN THE BEGINNING

Life is not a series of little sitcom episodes, quickly resolving with everyone living happily ever after. In a flash, peace takes flight and good times are eclipsed by bad news. And so it was with my life. In Houston, Texas, 1970, with lots of love, great friends, and family, Don and I started our life together. We had so much fun! We laughed a lot! When I got Don, I got his family too! I loved his mother, Gay, and she loved me like no one ever had. She was the first person, since my grandmother Elizabeth went to heaven, that showed me the unconditional love of God. She had a love for me that was unexplainable. She gave me a glimpse of the love of God. I also loved his family. When visiting Don's home in Virginia, we ate that good old homemade mountain dinners cooked by Gay and Aunt C. We explored the mountainside, walking where Don had played as a boy. Our get-togethers, with all the sisters, brothers, aunts, uncles, and cousins, were accompanied by lots of laughter as they each told stories of their life growing up in the hills of Virginia. Our best friends in Houston were Karen and Hubert. We made so many memories with them, dining in Houston's finest restaurants, traveling countless times to Las Vegas, and driving the Houston area countryside together. We still visit them and laugh about old times.

In 1972 we discovered we were going to have a baby and were delighted. As the baby grew inside my womb, something was happening deep in my soul. I knew there was more to life than just having a good time. My heart began to search for true meaning, stability, and security. One day I was walking outside. Suddenly I stopped and looked up into the sky. It's as if I could see God's panorama and His handwriting on the tables of heaven. Instantly I knew that if Don and I kept living the way we were, our family would end up like my family - torn apart by bitterness. I began to search for something more.

Church never worked for me. I had grown up with Churchianity, and it had not helped my family at all. The faith I grew up with was rule-based, cold, judgmental, and lifeless. There had been special moments when the life of God stirred in me. When I was about 7-years-old, my father was a deacon in our church. One of his responsibilities was to visit the 'shut-ins' with communion or The Lord's Supper, as they called it. The grape juice stood for the blood of Jesus, and the bread represented the body of Jesus. One night my whole family loaded up in the car, including my dad, mom, brother David, and sister, Honey (Alene). We went to visit one of the 'shut-ins.' Back in the day, shut-ins were confined due to a physical or mental disability and could not go to church. We arrived at the hospital. My family stayed in the car while my father and I went inside. My dad was so happy and full of love as he spoke words of encouragement to the frail, gray-haired lady. With gentle reverence, he served her The Lord's Supper, first the bread then the grape juice. Her tender smile revealed her gratitude as he prayed.

There were other memorable moments when Dad would join me on the piano bench. We would sing together in harmony as I played hymns. At other times my friend Olivia and I would practice singing hymns in her home as her mother led and coached us on the piano. Some Sunday evenings, Olivia and I would sing duets at her church where her mom was the music director. "Whispering Hope" was one of my favorite songs. My home was incredibly dysfunctional at that time, filled with conflict and sorrow. Sometimes, in despair, my heart would reach up for help, but there was none. The heavens seemed silent. My stretch upward did not reach far enough, nor was my cry loud enough. But God was building a powerful potential in me to brave the storms of life. I love Him for the route He planned for me in this life. My grandmother, Elizabeth, was full of love. She loved and needed God all her life. She was vulnerable yet resilient at the same time. Her heart contained a deep, quiet, peaceful stream that led to God. When I would visit her, we would go to tent revivals or go to her local country church that only met once a month because the preacher was a circuit rider. On Saturdays, she would pull her chair up close to the console radio and listen to Christian quartets.

Now I was grown, married, and going to have a baby. I was desperate for more. I did not know what that 'more' was, but my heart longed for it when I was by myself. I had tried Transcendental Meditation(TM). At that time, the Beatles had hit the shores of the United States. Their music captured the hearts of all the young people. They had a powerful, unique sound. They also spoke about their practice of TM. Meditating on a mantra was supposed to bring you peace and contentment. Always adventurous, my dad encouraged me to go to the TM center with him. He was also desperately searching for more than religion could offer. I received my mantra and gave TM a good try, but it left me empty. At the same time, Don and I were having lots of fun times. But I found that the joy of fun times was fleeting. I quickly identified with the song, *Good Time Charlie's Got The Blues.* Again I was left empty. I knew there had to be something more.

My mother and father moved from Houston to Indianapolis, Indiana due to a job transfer. They began calling and exclaiming that their life was changing. They believed they had found 'something more' through their relationship with Jesus Christ. They were both so happy and full of joy for the first time in their lives. I was delighted for them, but I was not sure that church life was for me. Because they were filled with new-found happiness, I thought maybe there was something to this Jesus thing. In my quiet time, I continued to yearn for more. I looked up beyond my own horizon like I had many times, searching for something more. I began to connect with the true and living God. I started having experiences with Him in my home. I had always believed that either He is real or not. If He is real, He can reveal himself to me personally and not through a church or religion.

Our first child Tim was born. I had never loved anything or anyone in my life like I loved my sweet baby, Tim. I was experiencing a portion of the love God feels for each of us. My relationship with the true and living God was blossoming. I began to read my Bible every day. I would wake up early to be alone with Him through His word and in contemplative prayer. One night when Don was away and Tim was fast asleep, I felt the urging of the Holy Spirit to get down on my knees beside my bed and pray. I had never prayed on my knees before. But like a little child, I obeyed God. I poured out my heart. My prayer was simple and child-like. 'Jesus, I'm scared. And I don't know what this commitment will bring. But I give my life completely to you.' I felt such peace, trust, and a sense of adventure. I had entered a new reality. God had taken my life. I was no longer in control. He was leading, and I happily followed.

Brian was born in 1976. What a delight he was! Don and I were happy with our two boys. I continued to get up early, spend time with God through His word and contemplative prayer. One day, when Brian was almost two years old, and Tim was five, I had to take the car to the dealership for a minor repair. I had no one to take me and drop me off. I knew I had a miserable morning ahead of me. I had to wait while the mechanic worked his magic with two small boys in tow. I had to stick around an hour or more in the dealership's filthy waiting room. I knew I had to change my attitude about the morning from dread to acceptance and peace. I had learned there was power in praise. Every time I grew impatient, I would praise the Lord in my heart. Through it all, trips to the bathroom, diaper changes, redirecting the boys, I celebrated the Lord in my heart. After a while, the wait was over. The car was ready, and we were on our way home.

As soon as we walked in the back door, I placed Brian in his baby bed. He was fast asleep. At the same time, Tim ran out of the front door to play.

All was quiet in the house - Whew! Suddenly I felt Holy Spirit say, 'Go to Brian's room and kneel in front of the rocking chair.' Again, kneeling to pray was not my usual prayer posture, but I obeyed. The voice was leading me with love and peace. I knelt and bowed my head. Then the Spirit of God began to lift my head, causing me to look upward as I prayed.

Suddenly a river of love began to flow from heaven to me, saturating my weary soul. The stream rushed back up to heaven, repeating its powerful pathway, over and over! I had never felt such love - the love and glory of God filled my being. The flow and flooding continued for a while, then stopped. I got up and walked out of Brian's room into the dining room. There was my Bible, open on the table. Until now, I had been faithfully reading His word and searching the scriptures. But something had changed. Suddenly, as I turned the pages, I realized I could understand the Bible like I never had before. I had been baptized, immersed in His Spirit. My eyes and heart were open in a new way.

God's Word filled me up, but my hunger for His words of life was more intense than ever. I was growing from a tender sprout to a tree full of fruit. I wanted to teach what I was learning. We started going to a local church that loved and cared for my family. I met with the pastor, Jim Ainsworth, and told him I would like to teach a ladies Bible study guided by Evelyn Christenson's book, *What Happens When Women Pray*. He agreed, and I began to teach. The Bible Study was a success. To this day, I still love to study and teach God's word. His word is new to me every day.

Our boys grew, and we enjoyed our time with them. We went through the challenges of a growing family and raising two boys. Don enjoyed great success in business and was a wonderful provider. When the boys reached their teens, I obtained a Masters Degree and became a Speech-Language Pathologist. I have also enjoyed many successful seasons in business. God was with us through joy in good times and the depths of grief in hard times. He strengthened our faith by what He taught us through it all! The boys left home and now have families of their own. We have four fabulous grandchildren that we love dearly. There is no greater joy than being a Grand to a Grand.

Chapter 2

MOVING FORWARD

In 1997 Don and I moved from the Houston area to Tyler, Texas. We joined a dynamic family of faith, Tyler Metro Church. Both of us continued to enjoy lots of success in business. In 2001 we moved to the Atlanta, Georgia area for about four years to be near Tim and his family. We continued to grow closer together, and our faith in God increased. We spent many weekends with Don's Virginia family. Mike, Wanda, Michelle, and Jason took us on many adventures through the mountains hiking, fishing, treasure-hunting, laughing all the way. We traveled to Florida to be with Don's Florida family. Don's sister Fonda and her husband Herb wowed us with their over-the-top Christmas decorations. We also spent many weekends traveling to various revivals - Calhoun, Georgia at a little Church of God, Bonnie and Mahesh Chavda, Charlotte, NC, Brownsville Revival, Pensacola, Florida. I am a revivalist at heart and love passionate encounters with God. Once you experience His love up close and personal, you are never the same.

We moved back to Tyler, Texas, where I worked for a home health agency for over seven years. Then I decided I wanted a change. My sister, Alene (Honey), moved from her position as a nurse with Texas Children's

Hospital to Texas Children's Health Plan as a Nurse Case Manager. She was training to work from home as a part of the remote work staff and told me about an open position for a speech-language pathologist. I applied for the job and got it. I would be training in Houston in the medical center for six months and then go back home to Tyler and work out of my home office. I moved in with my sister and her husband, Tom, in the Houston area during my training. We had great times together. Tom would laughingly introduce us as his sister wives. I would travel home or to the deer lease to meet Don on most weekends. Being away from him was one of the hardest things I had ever done. But all my life, God had put me in positions of distress to develop perseverance - the ability to move forward successfully, in the face of great pain, and endure to the end!

When I started my job in Houston with Texas Children's Health Plan as Utilization Management Speech Specialist, my sister was still in training. Our days were long and hard. Each morning we left her home in Spring at the crack of dawn and drove into the Houston Medical Center together. As only two sisters can, we chattered most of the way into Houston and back home in the evening. The real benefit she and I both had to look forward to was working from home. After about two months, she was able to go home and work. She had completed her six months of training. I was now traveling alone to Houston and back each day. Each trip along the teeming tollways and interstates was at least 70 nail-biting, white-knuckle ride, heart-pounding minutes. I dreaded every trip. It was tough being away from Don that long with only a few visits here and there, but we made it. I prayed a lot from deep within. One evening I was on my way home from work. I called Don each evening to check-in. I had just hung up from talking to him. I was on my freaky ride home to my sister's house.

Anguish was closing in on me at that moment. I realized Don needed me to be with him, and I was feeling the icy fear of knowing I could get killed any minute on those harrowing Houston roadways. I reached up to God from my heart and prayed one of those 'windshield prayers' with tears in my eyes. Jean's definition of a wind-shield prayer is a plea made when you are driving. Suddenly, you seize the steering wheel, reach up and grab heaven with your eyes and heart, and cry out to God from deep within. At that moment, through tears, I prayed, "God, please let me get home to take care of Don." Little did I know that soon, he would be taking care of me.

Near the end of February 2016, after six months of training, I arrived back home in Tyler. I set up all the equipment in our guest bedroom and converted it to an office. I happily began my life as a remote worker. My commute was easy. I would glide with my second coffee cup in hand down the hall of my home, log on, and start my day. Don would make and bring me breakfast. Lunch was easy. Just go to the refrigerator and look for leftovers. I took breaks frequently. I was happy to be home with Don. Our life was incredibly blessed.

Chapter 3

MANAGING HEALTH AND WELLNESS

One thing that had followed me from Houston to home was a nagging, chronic cough. I started having chest pains that would come and go. I did not tell Don, because I knew he would worry. One night I woke up with the chest pains and debated whether to awaken Don to take me to the ER or call 911 for an ambulance. I knew if it was my heart, I should contact 911, but I did not want to attract neighborhood drama with an ambulance siren sound in the middle of the night. So I did a dumb thing. I got up, packed my bag, just in case I had to go to the hospital, then went back to bed. The next day, working in my office, the cough and chest pains persisted. Having an incredible work ethic, I wanted to finish strong that day. As the afternoon progressed, the chest pains got worse. I was gripping my chest, bound and determined to finish my work. When I finished, about 5 PM, I told Don I was having chest pains and told him I thought it was a heart attack. I needed to go to the emergency room. After a long wait in the ER and several tests, they admitted me to the hospital with bilateral pneumonia. Who knew? Not me! I was healthy, ate right, exercised regularly, and took care of myself. I was surprised that my body had fallen prey to that diagnosis. I was in the hospital for two days. Then, after three days of rest at home, I was back to work in my comfortable home office with Don.

Now it was time for me to start the rounds of regular, preventative-care physician appointments I had put off for the last six months. So at the end of April, I went for a well-person check-up with my primary care physician. As a part of my examination that day, I had a routine mammogram. I checked that off my list of things to do as I rode back home and happily went back to work in my home office.

A few days later, I received a call from the East Texas Medical Center Breast Care Center in Tyler. The lady on the phone said there was a change in my mammogram findings in my right breast compared to the last reading and that my doctor wanted me to have a follow-up mammogram. She said not to worry too much. She explained that this was just a routine procedure. I scheduled my appointment for May 17th. I did not tell Don about it because I knew there was no need for alarm. After all, it had only been about a year and a half since my last mammogram. Besides, I had eaten very healthy food for more than a year-no sugar, lots of fresh vegetables, no highly refined carbohydrates, and quality protein.

On May 17, 2016, as I left home for my appointment for a follow-up mammogram, I had no clue my life would be changed forever that day. I submitted to the follow-up mammogram and dutifully returned to the waiting room while the radiologist studied the results. Then the nurse informed me that the doctor wanted to see me. Next, they wanted to do an ultrasound. They placed me in a separate room with the Diagnostic Radiologist, Dr. Klouda. He performed the ultrasound in silence. He kept going over certain spots and taking pictures. It was unnerving, but what was there to worry about? I had had an ultrasound of my breast many years ago. The diagnosis at that time was benign cysts from drinking too much caffeine. I continued pushing my encroaching, anxious thoughts to the side.

Abruptly Dr. Klouda broke his silence and said, "We look at your breast like the face of a clock. You have a tumor in your right breast at 12 o'clock and calcifications at 2 o'clock. I think it's cancer." What, me, cancer? Oh my, this can't be happening. I asked, "Why do you think it's cancer?" He responded, "Because of the shape of the tumor. Get dressed, and I'll meet you across the hall." I was stunned but not immobilized. There had to be some reasonable explanation for this. I think this is probably some kind of mistake.

I went across the hall with my life on pause. I was struggling to digest all of this, but my thinking was mushy and muddled. Questions were clashing in my head like indistinct symbols. My heart was racing. Soon Dr. Klouda appeared. He showed me the video of the ultrasound. He pointed out what he had seen, stopping and explaining at 12 o'clock and 2 o'clock. Again he said, "I think it's cancer." I was in disbelief and said, "Why do you think it's cancer?" He responded quietly and gently, "Because I have been doing this for over twenty years. The tumor is characteristic of ones that are cancerous, and the calcifications look like pre-cancerous calcium deposits. I want to schedule you for a biopsy of both the tumor and the calcifications." I looked at the screen. The calcium deposits looked like a constellation of stars. By this time, I was operating on autopilot. I was numb. I got dressed in silent slow motion. Then I scheduled the biopsy for May 25th, which seemed like forever away. Yet I was in no hurry at all.

Chapter 4

BEING BRAVE

To develop your bravery, you must stand up to something bigger than yourself. My 'something bigger' was on the doorstep knocking. On the way home, I objectively decided the next steps I needed to take. I say 'objectively' because there were two realities wrestling inside me - an eerie composure bordering on bone-chilling fear. I had to stay calm. The first thing I had to do was tell Don about the findings. He thought I had just gone for a routine doctor's appointment. I walked in the front door, greeted Don, and said, "There's something I have to tell you." I sat down on the couch as he sat in his chair. We were facing each other just like we did every day for our Bible study. I said, "I just got back from a follow-up mammogram. I have a tumor and calcifications in my right breast. They think it's cancer."

I tossed the words out of my mouth before I lost the nerve. Don just sat there on pause, not saying anything, much longer than the talkative Don ever goes without saying something. Suddenly all his questions started tumbling out. I answered them all with the meager but shocking information I had. Somewhere in the middle of that conversation, we both began to cry and embrace. We had been married for almost 46 years. We had experienced so much happiness together. We had also fought many battles, hand in hand, and won. In an instant, we knew that God would be with us each step of the way. Don said, "Everything is going to be alright. God will see us through. Let's pray." As we held each other tight, he prayed for our situation and put it in God's hands. I went back to work in my home office, knowing what the next two steps in this new reality had to be - call my two sons and tell them the news.

I was desperately calling on courage. In my home office, I began working. I proceeded to process this morning's events as best I could. I had entered a new state of being - completely healthy one minute then looking at the possibility of cancer the next. This uncertainty could not be real. But I knew I must continue to move forward and execute the following steps. As I thought about calling my sons with the news, tears began to well up in my eyes. My heart was stuck in my throat. Sons don't like to hear or see their mothers cry. I did not know if I could get the words out without breaking down. Intermittently Don would come back to the office and sit on the day bed. While experiencing his own disbelief and fear, he would assure me that everything would be alright and that we would get through this together.

Finally, I mustered up the courage to call my older son, Tim. I inhaled deeply, gathering all my strength so I would not break down and cry. When Tim answered, I greeted him. I haltingly told him I had some news. Then I explained all that I knew. He was surprised but calm in his response, asking a few questions. Then we were off the phone. I immediately broke down and cried. There is something about the relationship you have with your children that is so tender - like no other. A mom does not want to cause her children fear or grief, but I knew that truth, openness, and honesty are powerful. Families need to share joy, success, sorrow, disappointment, and pain. I knew that God was in control and would take care of all of us. Somehow I knew He would do something great in my children, down deep, through all of this. His undefinable mercy and grace always emerge when life's twists and turns have you submerged in deep waters. A shared crisis can break down unrealized, undefined barriers to the flow of love when you rally together to support one another.

Now I keep saying, 'I knew' as if I knew. But I didn't. I was walking in a foreign reality called uncertainty. I grabbed hold of God like a man grabs the tightrope he's been walking on as he falls toward the depths below. Life is unpredictable. In those times, when you feel like you are sinking, move toward the shoreline by holding on to God. Grab Him and hold on with all the strength and courage you have. Don't worry about what you don't have. He will give you what you lack.

Now it was time to call Brian. I continued to work at my desk and reach deep within for the peace to call Brian. I did not want to break down, but I was on the verge. Then I placed the call. I sounded calm as I told him the news. I answered the questions he asked and was soon off the phone. I again broke down and cried like a baby. When I gained my composure, I called my sister, Alene. She was so supportive. A few years ago, she had experienced her own cancer diagnosis and subsequent grueling treatment. She had moved through the anguishing fear, the complex medical regimen that included debilitation, to complete health. Her words were calm and reassuring. She knew what I was going through.

Chapter 5

UNCERTAIN TESTING TIMES

On May 25th, I went for a breast biopsy. They took a tissue sample of the tumor at 12 o'clock but could not do the biopsy on the constellation of calcifications because their equipment was not working. Dr. Klouda asked if I remembered what we had discussed. I confirmed that I recalled he had said it was probably cancer. I questioned whether he still thought it was, and he said, "Yes." I asked about coming back for the biopsy of the calcifications. He responded as if it didn't matter. I think he knew my diagnosis would lead to mastectomy. He disclosed that his wife had experienced breast cancer. We discussed options for physicians. He said her surgeon was Dr. Fender, the one we eventually chose. On May 26th, I received the biopsy report - Grade 1, Stage 1, Multifocal, Invasive Ductal Cancer. Dr. Klouda explained that 'invasive' means the cancerous cells had broken out of the duct where it started and invaded the breast tissue. He elaborated that it predictably travels to the lymph nodes next. He said there was no evidence right now that the cancer cells had wandered.

We began our walk through the Land of Uncertainty. I say 'our walk' because Don traveled with me 'step for step'. We each had our separate walk, also. I'll share some of that with you as we move along the highway in this foreign territory. We began our journey with prayer putting our trust in God. We also committed ourselves and our mountain of need to our local family of faith, Tyler Metro Church. Immediately they started walking with us. We received personal prayer and corporate prayer. Often friends would let us know they were praying personally for us. There were days, moments, when I could feel someone praying me upward - days when I felt my own emotions were grounding any of my prayer efforts to get to God in the heavenly realm! I had started a journal with 'Word of God and Friend' entries to fight the battle. My journaling began May 31st:

Jesus Christ is the same yesterday, today, and forever.
From Hebrews 13:8 NKJV

Tearing down barriers erected against the truth of God, fitting every loose thought and emotion and impulse into the structure of life shaped by Christ.
From 2 Corinthians 10:5 MSG

For I will restore health to you and heal you of your wounds.
From Jeremiah 30:17 NKJV.

Call those things that do not exist as though they did.
From Romans 4:17 NKJV.

Having done all, to stand.
From Ephesians 6:13 NKJV.

I take hold of your strength.
From Isaiah 27:5 NKJV.

Jesus told the leper, Of course, I am willing to heal you, and now you will be healed.
From Luke 5:13 TPT.

So now we must cling tightly to the hope that lives within us, knowing that God always keeps His promises.
From Hebrews 10:23 TPT.

You will be satisfied with a full life and with all that I do for you. For you will enjoy the fullness of my salvation.
From Psalm 91:16 TPT.

I have come to give you everything in abundance, more than you expect-life and its fullness until you overflow.
From John 10:10 TPT.

I stood on His word. His word held me up like a scaffold. In some moments, His word was all I had and everything I needed. But I always needed more. I wanted to be healthy NOW and not go through the valley of the shadow! Don and I prayed. Our family and church prayed.

Chapter 6

FAVORABLE ENCOUNTERS AND CHOICES

We did not yet know what doctors we wanted to choose or where we wanted to go for treatment. We considered M. D. Anderson in Houston, Texas, a leading cancer center in the U.S. However, I was not sure I wanted to be in the Houston Medical Center with so much traffic and so far away from our children and my sister. I knew Don and I would need emotional and physical support. I also knew our family might want us to be near them so they could help. Although my son Brian and sister lived outside of Houston, I knew what a daring drive it would be to get from their homes to the Medical Center and so inconvenient to their schedules. Don and I prayed! We needed to choose the best medical care. We prayed every day for God's direction. Don has always carried the weight of our family. I could see that he was carrying the weight of this health crisis as well. One day, June 16, 2016, Don announced he was going to get a pedicure. I had been reminding him to go for weeks. The sudden decision to get a pedicure that particular day was unusual. When Don got back home, he was so happy. He sat on the daybed in my office and excitedly began to tell me about his visit. With his feet in the warm, swirling water, he shared our situation with Taylor, who had done our nails for years. A woman was getting her nails done at the same time. Don is not known for having a quiet voice. He learned to whisper in a sawmill. The lady heard every word. While Don was still seated, she started to leave. She slowly turned around and said, "I probably should not be saying anything, but I feel like I should. Within the last year, I was diagnosed with breast cancer. I stayed right here in Tyler for my treatment. I had a mastectomy with chemotherapy, radiation, and reconstruction right here in Tyler. You can get the same treatment here that you would get at M. D. Anderson Cancer Center. My doctors were Fender, Breast Surgeon, Harrison, Plastic Surgeon, and Usrey, Oncologist. They are the best!" Don asked her a few questions and was satisfied with the answers she gave. As Don sat on the daybed relaying this encounter to me, I could see that the burden of selecting physicians had been lifted off his shoulders. His spirit was so light and joyful. He believed this was God's pathway for us. I agreed that God was directing our path. Within a few days, I received a message from an old friend asking me to call her. She said she had read about my diagnosis on Facebook. She had some information to share. When I called, she told me she worked for an oncology group and recommended Dr. Fender, surgeon, Dr. Harrison, Plastic Surgeon, and Dr. Usrey, Oncologist. She advised that we did not need to go to M. D. Anderson. She explained that many people from the East Texas area who go to M. D. Anderson for consultation come back to Tyler for treatment. Don and I agreed that this was the answer.

> *Trust God from the bottom of your heart. Don't try to figure out everything on your own. Listen for God's voice in everything you do, everywhere you go. He's the one who will keep you on track.* From Proverbs 3:5, 6 MSG.

It was a great relief for us just to have made that decision. We had already chosen Dr. Fender as our surgeon due to Dr. Klouda's recommendation. Now we were waiting on a phone call for a consultation with Dr. Fender. And we waited and waited what seemed like an eternity for him to come back from vacation. You see, in the Land of Uncertainty, waiting one moment is eternally long. You long to return to the Land of Certainty where the pathway is clear, where there is no fear. In the Land of Certainty, you are in control. There $2 + 2 = 4$ and everything is predictable. You are living in Happily Ever After Land. I had counseled and taught others the word of God! I had attended church regularly and believed God was blessing our lives. I had memorized God's word. I had prayed for years and regularly prayed. My husband and I had regular Bible studies together. Suddenly "Wham!" Uncertainty with his ugly companion, Fear, had entered our lives.

In the meantime, I was gathering resources. I spoke with people who had been diagnosed with breast cancer and had finished their treatment. I found that each breast cancer diagnosis is unique. It comes to people of diverse backgrounds, different life circumstances, and all ages. It is certainly no respecter of persons. It also occurs in men, although it is rare. I learned about distinct courses of treatment for different diagnoses. I gathered information about medical treatment options and holistic treatment alternatives. On May 20, 2016, my sister in law, Wanda, connected me with a video series called The Truth About Cancer: A Global Quest hosted by Ty Bolinger. The nine-episode series gave me information about cancer from prevention to diagnosis to treatment options. I learned healthy alternatives or complementary therapies for cancer treatment.

In my search for information, I learned that people diagnosed with cancer loved to support others. When we connected, we could become fast friends in no time. One of Tim's friends heard about my diagnosis and told him she would be available to support me. On May 31, 2016, she told me her story. She had been diagnosed with breast cancer about a year before. Her cancer was Stage 3, Triple Negative. Triple-negative breast cancer is a subset of breast cancers that are not driven by estrogen or progesterone hormones. They also do not overexpress the HER-2/neu protein. Biologically, HER-2 is very aggressive and can grow more rapidly than other types of breast cancer. She sought her first opinion from an oncologist in Tyler who recommended a mastectomy, chemotherapy, then radiation, in that order. She then went to M. D. Anderson Cancer Center in Houston for a second opinion. They recommended chemotherapy, mastectomy, then radiation - different steps, same treatment. She chose to take chemotherapy in Tyler, have her mastectomy in Houston at M. D. Anderson, then radiation in Houston. She told me that her physician had recommended supplementation with Vitamin D 3 because studies had shown that people with low levels of Vitamin D were more likely to develop cancer. She gave me two books with information about what to eat and how the things you eat can be related to the cancer journey. I learned how to support healing through what I ate. The resources were *The Whole-Food Guide for Breast Cancer Survivors - A Nutritional Approach to Prevent Recurrence*, by Edward Bauman, Med, Ph.D. and Helayne Waldman, MS, EDD and *Foods to Fight Cancer - Essential Foods to Prevent Cancer*, by Richard Beliveau, Ph.D. and Denis Gingras, Ph.D.

A whole new world was opening up to me! I learned I had choices about my healthcare. I could choose my own treatment providers and treatment plan. I found that supplementation may help prevent a recurrence. I learned that food could become part of my treatment program. All were choices I could make. You see, this C diagnosis spins you around like a top until you are so dizzy you can hardly think straight. You feel totally out of control. You are in a strange territory! The doctors were familiar with all of the medical terms, crazy emotions, and swelling fears. But I was not. All of this was unknown to me. I was flung like a foreign body into outer space. Objects were coming toward me like a meteor shower at such speed that I could not make them out until they were past me. The language was different. An alien force had invaded my body. At times I felt like a boat that had slipped its mooring and was now adrift. I was fighting to maintain control and get some traction in this new terrain.

Chapter 7

BRAVE NEW WORLD

The diagnosis had knocked me down but not out. With each new piece of information, I was getting back up and in control, making informed choices. In partnership, God and I could maneuver this vessel safely to shore. Everything in my life began to look different. Instead of casting gloom, the disruption brought new life. This may sound totally off the chain to some, but all of nature was singing. The sky was bluer, the leaves were greener, the flowers more glorious. How could this be, right in the midst of one of the most overwhelming disturbances of my life? I felt like all things were new! Don't ask me why. I just did. I decided I wanted to be baptized again, so I was.

> *Now if anyone is enfolded in Christ, he has become an entirely new creation. All that is related to the old order has vanished. Behold, everything is fresh and new.*
> From 2 Corinthians 5:17 TPT.

I believe we should be in a constant state of revitalization. You may be molting like a bird losing its feathers, but soon you'll be sporting those stunning, new plumes. God wants to renew us day by day. He wants us to see His kingdom come, and His will be done in our spirit, soul, body, home, and all relationships. He wants us to become what He originally created us to be. Calamity can bring you to a crisis of faith where you are crumbled to bits like Humpty Dumpty. Then God begins to put you back together according to His design and for His glory. You can go from good to great. Only He can do that as we look to Him when things in our lives are turned upside down. Disruption is a business term where a radical change suddenly comes to an industry or business strategy. When disruption arrives, a business cannot continue using the same tools and methods, although they have been using them successfully for many years. If the market is to survive and advance, new ideas, tactics, techniques, products must be introduced, or the business will fade away. Disruption comes to our lives to make us stand up and pay attention. Assess the old, consider the new! Make a choice!

Sometimes we have to let go of the past before we can see the future - take a leap of faith! Some disruptions force that leap in the face of fear. Some people are immobilized and perplexed. They fear the loss of the familiar. They mourn the loss of past successes. They can't consider a new, better reality, even though God wants to give it to them. They are blinded by and chained to their previous successes or failures. Fear keeps their feet nailed to the floor so they can't move forward. They are stuck in the present even though all of life is moving on without them. The train has left the station, and all they can do is gaze at the caboose as it rumbles out of sight. They continue to exist in status quo or loss until they pass from this life to the next. No. God wants to make all things new in your life and my life. Be ready each day to think and embrace a way you have not yet imagined. He is waiting for you to look up.

So I held my head high and looked beyond my field of vision. My research led me to understand some of the possible causes of cancer. The first thing I decided to do was reduce my toxic load. Toxic load refers to the accumulation of toxins and chemicals in our bodies that we take in from various sources, including the environment, the food we eat, the water we drink, the personal care products we put on our body, and the household products we use. I learned that many things we breathe, put on our bodies, and put in our bodies contain toxins. I knew I could not avoid toxins altogether because of the world we live in, but I could at least take a step toward reducing the toxins I put on and in my body. My research led me to understand that many of the products I was putting on my body contained toxins and known carcinogens. For many years, I had used the most expensive makeup and face creams to keep myself younger. I had laughingly told Don several years ago that I will never retire because I want to continue to purchase expensive face care products to keep me young. Yikes! I was so wrong. I looked at the ingredients in the skin care line I was using and found it contained known carcinogens! I threw away a lot of expensive face cream. It didn't hurt nearly as bad as it could have, because I began to search for natural skincare options. I quickly learned that I could make my own. Amid the crucible, my mind was opened to novel ideas.

With great gusto, I developed natural skin care recipes and tried them on myself. If they did not work, I refined them or developed others. After I felt I had a pretty good product, I would ask my family to try them, asking for their feedback. I am proud to say I have developed my own product line called "Well Within." My family, including my son Tim, begs for more when he and his wife, Melissa, run out. Some friends buy the face scrub, my signature product, by the case (not expensive). It contains frankincense and myrrh, and both have anti-aging, life-giving properties for your skin and body. Some people use the face scrub on their animals, including dogs and horses. I am so proud God has led me to a new business. Although I still work full time for Texas Children's Health Plan, I have so many God ideas that I can't possibly pursue them all at once. He has unlimited creative ideas and opportunities waiting for you. He just wants you to look up.

Michelle, my niece, sent a powerful book, *Switch on Your Brain*, by Dr. Caroline Leaf. I learned that thoughts could be threatening or life-giving. Dr. Leaf documented research in neuroscience, concluding that as we think and imagine, we change the brain's structure. (Dr. Eric R. Kandel, Nobel

Prize-winning neuropsychiatrist p. 32). I learned that toxic thinking could negatively impact my DNA and that positive thoughts could have a life-giving effect on my DNA. I followed Dr. Leaf's 21-day brain detox plan. My mental and emotional resilience in the face of darkness grew. I developed a method to detox my thought-life, bringing a life-giving force to each new day. I continued my research in the field of neuroscience on thoughts and how they affect your body. Out of my research, I developed a plan to share with others. I started writing my book, *Mindful Meditation: 30 Days Uniting With the Heart of God*. It's now published and available on Amazon.

Chapter 8

MEDICAL MYSTERY TOUR

Finally, on June 15th, the day came when Don and I met with Dr. Fender, the breast surgeon. I never thought I would be walking this unsettling route with multiple bumps, twists, and turns. We were offered several options. Our final decision was bilateral, skin-sparing mastectomy with immediate reconstruction. Dr. Fender explained that they would also do a sentinel node biopsy just before surgery. In a sentinel node biopsy, they trace the sentinel lymph nodes (first drainage lymph node from the tumor) from the cancerous tumor to see if cancer has spread to the lymph nodes. I felt good about our decision, as good as a person could feel in this situation. My definition of normal was being discarded. We were following the path we believed God had laid out for us.

The next step was to visit Dr. Harrison, the plastic surgeon. Here we were again in the Land of Uncertainty - waiting. Dr. Harrison was on vacation. The Waiting Zone in the Land of Uncertainty is where Fear talks loud. Fear also knows how to create pictures of possibilities you don't want to see. You sit watching the Possibility Movies with one eye open and the other covered as Fear plays a horror show dramatizing where he says you are going. We could not get an appointment with Dr. Harrison until July 11th.

You've got to be kidding. Waiting a month was very hard. But it gave me time to strengthen my grip on the tightrope - time to secure my connection with God and His word. I needed that time because I was entering the territory called Crisis of Faith.

Finally the week came when we were to meet with Dr. Harrison, the plastic surgeon. Happily, this was also the week my grandson, River, came from Houston to spend time with us. Andrew, another grandson, also came to stay. We had such fun that week, laughing, playing, building bonfires, making bow and arrows, and dancing together! We gathered 'survival equipment' and put up a tent in the back yard. The boys wanted to spend the week in the tent and see if they could survive on very few resources. Of course, they loaded the tent with candy, crackers, cookies - survival food of choice for two eleven-year-old boys.

Thursday of that week, Don and I met with Dr. Harrison. The meeting was a real trip, the moment in time when reality began to set in. He painted a vivid picture of what they would do to my body. I remember things like - hollow your breast out like a pumpkin, one or both breast, cosmetic outcome, no nipples, temporary expanders, implants, drains. I sat in shock and wanted to run away. But I had to stay, trapped in a new existence. This sculpture was my twisted Picasso. As Dr. Harrison talked, bone-chilling fear would hit me in waves. At times I wanted to fall apart. Then Dr. Harrison would call me back to the present moment with a joke or a diversionary thought. I was crying one moment and laughing the next. He is so much fun yet filled with passion and compassion for people. He was one of our most staunch supporters.

I will never forget that day. We sat in his office for at least two hours as he explained the procedure and comforted us. But still, I was in walking shock - wading mentally and emotionally through quicksand. After we finish our visit, the next step was to check out at the front desk and plan the surgery. Tonia, his assistant, looked at my chart and said, "So you are going to have a bilateral mastectomy….." That's all I could hear. I felt like a gong had gone off in my soul. I was spinning inside. My logic pills weren't working. Everything was going dark. I spit out, "What? Did we agree to that?" I looked at her and then my husband. She got Dr. Harrison. Yes, I had agreed to that, but the words were cold, chilling, numbing, and much too real. Yes, that is what we had decided, but now things were sinking in. Dr. Harrison came back and reviewed what we had considered. I knew it was true, but I was grasping for stability. I will never forget that moment as long as I live. Talk about turmoil. I felt like a bomb had exploded in my back yard.

Thank God for an agile mind. I started exercising my mental muscles. I was able to pull myself up and out with God's help. I began to seek God and meditate on His word like never before. You see, we go THROUGH the Valley of the Shadow. We go THROUGH a Crisis of Faith. Unraveling is real, and you have to deal with what is for a while. A while means as long as it takes. We grow and go from glory to glory, from faith to faith. We must go through the process. We take leaps of faith during a crisis, not knowing how things are going to turn out. The blows were falling by degrees, giving me time to face it. God was leading me on a faith journey.

I was glad River and Andrew, two of our grandsons, were spending a few days with us. That night we had a bonfire and roasted marshmallows. We cranked up the music real loud and danced. They taught me how to do 'The Dab.' That's a dance, for those of you who may not know. We told stories, read books, and partied hardy that night. They brought me such joy. By the way, I can still do 'The Dab.'

Chapter 9

NEW REALITY

Something happened to me along the way that is difficult to understand and explain. I had entered a reality that was surreal yet very real. I was trusting God with everything in me. He was becoming my all-in-all. One day I was driving down the road, and suddenly my senses were keenly aroused. The sky had never been so bright and blue. I beheld the beauty and majesty of the trees like never before. The birds never sang so sweetly. The sun never shined so brightly. My heart was singing in tune with nature. My emotions were on alert as I cried readily and laughed spontaneously. That intensity is still with me today. I love with much more purpose and intent than ever before.

On July 19th, I spoke with a representative at Dr. Fender's office. My surgery was scheduled for August 2nd. I was to arrive at 6 AM for the nuclear, sentinel node injection for mapping and biopsy. The time of surgery was 11:15 AM. Fender's part of the operation, breast removal, and the removal of four lymph nodes were to take two hours. Then Harrison would begin breast reconstruction, adding the expanders. Dual reality again came to play. I was living through the stark, naked circumstances of my life.

Yet God was comforting me! That day I wrote in my journal, 'I feel a new beginning coming on. He is making all things new. God is renewing us all like springtime. And we didn't even know we had been living in winter. Behold He makes all things new!' God's active word was birthed in the silence of my soul. On July 20, 2016, I wrote:

> Grace is flowing amid troubled waters.
> Power is rising out of the storm.
> All things are new!
> Who had a clue?
> That joy could be so great,
> Crushing doom and gloom!

That evening, after nearly forty years, I was rebaptized, this time by our Pastor, Dr. Jerry Phelps. God was changing everything, and all of life was new. My meditation became His word. Joy filled my heart. God's enemies were scattering like mice fleeing a stalking cat. God gets up when He's had enough. Enough is enough.

> *You will arise and have mercy on me.*
> From Psalm 102:13 NKJV.

> *For the time to favor me, yes, the set time has come. God will regard the prayers of the destitute.*
> From Psalm 102:17 NKJV.

> *Joseph was sold into Egypt, but God was with him and delivered him out of all his troubles and gave him favor and wisdom in the presence of those in power.*
> From Acts 7:9 NKJV.

Now the surreal was merging with reality. On July 25, 2016, I was planning time away from work following surgery. I notified my boss and Human Resources about my medical condition. I applied for time away for surgery and recovery with the Family Medical Leave Act (FMLA). However, I was not yet eligible for that benefit, because I had not worked for the company a year. I did qualified for another benefit, similar to FMLA. I calculated the days off I had earned, including PTO and Emergency Illness Bank. I discussed with my physician the time I would need to recuperate before returning to work. I was dealing with the realities of life and planning for an uncertain future. My meditation that day:

He will call upon me, and I will answer him in trouble and distress. I will rescue him and honor him. With long life, I will satisfy him and show him my salvation.
From Psalm 91:15, 16 NKJV.

Chapter 10

FACING THE GIANTS

There's pain that uses you and pain that you use. I was using pain to push me forward. One of the first things I had to do was confront the possibility of death. That specter rose his ugly head every single day, several times a day of my faith odyssey. I knew God has something to say about everything, including death. So I studied God's word. I was walking through the Valley of the Shadow of Death. According to Psalms 23, I could decide to fear no evil. I had been at the bedside of many who had passed from this life to the next. I saw how easy it was for them to transition. At that moment, light and glory filled the room as their body was released from all struggles. Their spirit had 'left the building.' They were no longer a part of this present reality. After the death of my grandmother in 1974, I wanted to discover what death was. My mother, Rachel, had become a Christian and wanted to know what God, medical science, and people with near-death experiences had to say about death. I became a student with her and still have some of the books we studied. I pulled them off the shelf and read them again. I looked at God's word and found sustaining stability. Paul, the apostle, faced death many times. Paul said,

> We are convinced that even if these bodies of ours are folded up at death like tents, we will still have a God-built home that no human hands have built, which will last forever in the heavenly realm.
> From 2 Corinthians 5: 1 TPT.

I found that if I died, I would be moving from my present body to a body prepared by God. One day it will be moving day for each of us. All that I read about death comforted me, including the dying process and transitioning from this life to the next. But I was not ready for the move. I was crying out to God like the psalmist,

> Father of eternity, please don't let me die. I know my life is not yet finished.
> From Psalms 102:24 TPT.

I also had questions like 'why me.' I had great faith in God, studied and taught His word, ate right, lived a life of forgiveness, etc. How did this happen to me? I have met so many people with a cancer diagnosis that said the same thing. "I have been a vegan for ten years and eaten only organic food." "I was a marathon runner and ate all the right things." "I was a bicycler and taught martial arts." Everybody has their own way of maintaining good health, trying to ward off a health crisis. You will never get the answer to 'Why.'

I devoured the book my friend Karen sent me by Bob Sorge, *Pain, Perplexity, and Promotion*. I meditated on each chapter. I was in pain and mental anguish. I was perplexed - stunned and unprepared for this episode of my life. I had always yearned for promotion in His Kingdom - more intimacy with God and empowerment to take God's good news to others. But not this way. Karen and I talked several times a week. She would always point me upward toward the prize. My questions turned into a step forward, "God, I want to know You more. I want to walk in the land You have prepared for me. I want to walk this out with You." God has an adventure awaiting all of us. Sometimes the prize is in disguise. The wrapping paper is rumpled. The package is bland and bowless. You dare not open it alone.

Like a baby chick inside an egg, you must peck your way out to a brand new world.

You don't know how things are going to turn out. You pray, develop your faith, ask God for a miracle, and trust Him through the process to the end. Either way, you win. Continue to travel this life in your earth suit or go home to be with Him in your glorified body.

We are a colony of heaven on earth as we cling tightly to our life-giver, the Lord Jesus Christ, who will transform our humble bodies, and transfigure us into the identical likeness of His glorified body. Using His matchless power, He continually subdues everything to Himself.
From Philippians 3: 20, 21 TPT.

What about faith and miracles? I have grown enough in my faith to know that God is working in all things, good and bad. And He is working all things for my good. Sometimes we hear reports that someone has a diagnosis of doom. Then someone prays. Then they go back to the physician, and the sickness is gone. People will say, "God heard your prayers." or "What a miracle!" But what about those of us that have to walk it out? Some of us are walking through the Valley of the Shadow. What about people that die? God is still working miracles in the dark, in your heart, that no man can see. For one person, the gift may be a more profound love for others. For another, it may be greater faith. We all walk our own pathway. We all have our own race to run. We can't say that God is with those who are healed, but He has fallen off the throne when they are not made healthy or die. Trust is a little five-letter word, but it is boundless to God. He wants us to trust Him and Him alone. We must all choose our pathway to well-being and health. Another should not judge the path we choose. There were many moments I had to throw myself into His arms. I was weak, but He was strong. He wove great things into my being as I learned to trust Him more. My faith muscles got an intense workout. I stepped it out daily with Him. My trust-potential grew, and I learned to stroll with Him shoulder-to-shoulder.

My friend Georgia, a counselor who had also walked through the same diagnosis, gave me some great advice. "Give yourself permission and time to grieve." She knew me well. She knew I could easily mask my feelings, bury them, and then walk on like everything was fine. I was skilled at minimizing pain. I had learned to do that as a child, hounded by unrelenting disappointment, sorrow, and unchanged circumstances. I knew Georgia's recommendation was wise counsel and I needed to take heed. She knew God wanted to work deep in my heart. As we were talking, another well-meaning friend passed by saying, "Get another scan. God has healed you." Georgia said, "How did that make you feel?" I replied, "Intimidated, afraid, threatened, not able to own my emotions, not free to walk out my own pathway to healing." I knew to spring back and not shrink back. I wanted to be authentic, vulnerable, and open with people and with God. I wanted to be honest and free with my Rock and my Redeemer. He is my Heavenly Father. He knows me better than and loves me more than anyone. Georgia reported that when she told her friends about her diagnosis, many said things like, "Oh, that's okay. You'll be fine." She explained that they bypassed her emotional responses, not allowing her to have emotions - to be afraid, to grieve the loss of....

I have spoken with several friends who had been diagnosed with breast cancer. Some had a lumpectomy with radiation. One is still bearing the physical scars, the change in typography and texture, and extreme sensitivity when she accidentally bumps that breast. Another was soon divorced. Yet all are moving forward, living life with great gusto, smiling because it happened and changed their lives.

Chapter 11

CELEBRATION OF LIFE

What do you do the night before you go to war? Celebrate, laugh, talk about yesterday, and look toward a great tomorrow. August 1, 2016, the day before my 'unbreasting' was quite eventful. My surgery was initially scheduled for July 21st. However, due to physician scheduling changes, it was delayed. By this time, I was good at waiting. Not really. The celebration of life began the night before surgery when our friends, Karen and Hubert, arrived from Navasota, Texas. My sister, Alene, came from Burton, Texas. Because Alene was a nurse and my sister, I wanted her with me, close by, all the time. I love her so much, and she and I have promised each other to help during times like this. We always have and always will. We all gathered at my home with my son Tim and his family. We celebrated family, friendship, and the closeness we all shared.

Then everyone said their good-byes, going home or to their hotel rooms, except Alene. She helped me follow pre-op instructions that night. We talked it all through. Then it was time for us to get some rest. Surgery time would come early the next morning. All alone, through my tears, I looked at my breasted body for one of the last times. It was a bitter-sweet moment. On my breasts, I had born deep emotions like love and sensual feelings. I had lovingly nursed my babies. I wondered, 'Will I still love with the same intensity?' I wanted to continue feeling whole, both physically and emotionally.

Chapter 12

GAME DAY

August 2, 2016, Don, Alene, and I got up before dawn. With Alene's help, I did my final at-home pre-surgical prep. It was now time to go to the hospital. The sun was beginning to rise. The flow of traffic was more substantial than usual. All hospital staff was changing shifts. I remember the ride well and how hard it was for me - agonizing. I struggled to keep myself together-breathing deeply, fighting back the tears. When we arrived at the hospital, I checked in and waited for the next step, engaging in trivial small-talk with my sister while Don parked the car. Next they took me to what I later named 'the holding pen'. I was to gown up and get in bed. Again, I was waiting. I hate that 'w' word, where seconds saunter slowly like snails in a garden. Don't these people know this is torture? Give me some happy medicine and put me out of my misery. But no, with them it's first things first.

The medical theater was buzzing with practiced precision movement. The nurses started wiping me down, preparing for the sentinel node tracing. I insisted my sister go with me. Don stayed in the waiting room, nervously anticipating the events of the day. By this time, a host of friends and family were arriving, and they were a great comfort to him. Alene accompanied me as I was rolled in the wheelchair to the sentinel node injection area - one last insult to the breast before they remove it. I knew this was a necessary step. Sentinel lymph node mapping and biopsy are the best way to determine if breast cancer cells have escaped the original tumor and spread to nearby lymph nodes in the armpit. This procedure's location was the same place where I had first heard the words 'I think it's cancer' following the mammogram. The same place where they did the biopsy and again said, 'I think it's cancer.' And now - Oh my God, another insult to my body and emotions. Doesn't anybody see? I'm just barely holding myself together here! We arrived for the injection. I changed into my robe and asked that my sister accompany me for the procedure. The nurse seemed reluctant and explained that the doctor did not like anybody else in the room. I wanted my sister with me, and I was on the verge of insisting when the young lady said she would ask the doctor if it was alright. She returned, saying the doctor agreed. Alene and I slowly went into the room, and I lay down on the table - waiting again. Really? Are you kidding me?

I had been told by a friend previously diagnosed with breast cancer with mastectomy following that the sentinel node biopsy was the worst part and that the experience was harrowing. I was not looking forward to a needle gouging my breast. When Dr. Klouda, the Diagnostic Radiologist, arrived, I was lying there ready to get the show on the road, thankful that my sister was in the room. He silently began his preparation. In my heart, I'm praying and distracting myself from fear with praise. I wanted to run away, but the doctor broke his silence and began his verbal guidance, explaining what he was doing each step of the way. Then it was over. No pain. No trauma. I was so thankful I had not felt a thing that I almost kissed the doctor. Thank God that step was behind me. Then back to the holding pen before going into surgery.

As I lay on the hospital bed, next to the surgical suite, in my hospital gown with white curtains surrounding me before surgery (with no happy medicine, I might add), God did great things. A great glory filled the room as friend-after-friend and family-member after family-member came to see me one or two at a time. Two was the hospital limit. Each spoke beautiful words of life and prayed with me. I cannot possibly explain the joy and glory that filled that room. It must have filled the whole waiting room. Soon Don was directing traffic from the waiting room to the holding pen. The nurses gave him the run of the place. He would bring two people to see me then get others. We had such a wonderful time. One at a time, my anesthesiologist, breast surgeon, and plastic surgeon all came to see me, gave me a greeting with last-minute instructions, then prayed with me. What a God-filled time it was. Then it was surgery time. Happy medicine would take me to another world.

And I don't remember another thing until I woke up in the recovery room. I looked around, and everything seemed light, bright, white. I lifted my head and said, "Where am I?" My plastic surgeon, Dr. Harrison, spoke with ethereal drama in his deep voice from behind the desk, "You're in Heaven!" What a sense of timing that man has! That made me laugh! In a timeless world, I moved in and out of a peaceful dream state. Then they announced my room was ready. God's feeling of glory and love was still on me. Yes, I know I had lots of joy juice in my system too. I could feel the love of God. Melissa, my daughter in law, said I held her hand the whole way on the ride. I was riding on the gurney, feeling no pain. Don, Tim, Melissa, and Alene were walking and talking all around me. Quite an entourage. The nurse must have been directing the parade, but somehow he was silent. No other word can force entry into a Winebarger gabfest unless you are given the floor. Apparently, in that inebriated state, I told my son Tim that he should look at the surgical area of my chest. Tim can barely stand the sight of any kind of blood. I was horrified later when they told me about it. At that time, I was not even brave enough to look at myself. My valiant spirit was playing hide-and-seek. I did not want to see.

My sister spent the night making sure the staff took good care of me. Nurses drifted in and out of my room that night. Dr. Harrison arrived at the hospital before daylight the next morning to check on me. He removed the bandages. For the first time, I was forced to see my chest 'unbreasted.' The pain meds took the edge off of the first viewing. I knew I had to face this topographical change in my body. So I forced myself each day to bravely embrace the stark alteration, being thankful in all and for all.

Chapter 13

RECOVERY ROAD

I will spare you the details of recovery from surgery. To put it mildly, it was difficult. The pain pills, my sweet husband, my sister's help, a beautiful family, and my loving church family made it so much easier. My friend Lou Ann arranged for many friends from the church to bring dinner to us every other day for over two weeks. The food was delicious but more precious than the meals were the sweet visits we had with each one. They will never know just how much their presence and their words of comfort meant to Don and I. We gathered strength from each one. My sister helped with the medical care during my recovery until I got strong enough, and Don was confident he could do it. Tim, Melissa, Addison, Emma, and Andrew would visit almost every day, sharing their love and the fantastic food we had leftover. I thank God for a family of love and faithfulness!

Was it good news or bad news? At first, immediately following surgery, the physician told Don everything was fine. He did not think cancer had spread. They explained that the final report would come from the pathologist in a few days. Then Dr. Fender called two days after surgery. Of the four sentinel lymph nodes they had mapped and removed, two nodes contained lobular carcinoma. Of the two nodes with lobular cancer, one was of a different histology or shape-pleomorphic. He explained that only 5% of lobular carcinomas are pleomorphic, 'so we don't know much about it.'

The news about the nodes was, to say the least, unsettling. What did all that mean? Fear tried to creep in. I was fighting it off as best I could. Uncertainty was my new normal. All I could do was hold on one minute, one hour, one day at a time. I fought to shift my mind and heart to God's word, knowing all things work together for good to those that love God and are called to fulfill His purposes. I knew nothing could separate me from His love, and that fear cannot stand in the face of perfect love. I began to seek the love of God more than ever. God is love. I was seeking His presence in my life and heart more and more. I also yearned for that love to flow through me to others. I knew that love is a life-giving force that can fill your being and bring change.

On August 8, 2016, Don and I quietly celebrated our 46th wedding anniversary at home. I was still recovering, and we were happy to be together. We reviewed our history as a couple, telling old stories again. When we married, we knew it would be forever. But we never thought we'd be married 46 years. When we married, we didn't have any idea what 46 years meant. I was 22, and he was 31 years old. We had not yet even lived for 46 years. I wrote in my journal that day, "I feel as though God is carving me out, gutted from deep within so that He can pour in something great - something that could not be discovered or poured out otherwise." My friend, Karen, called that day. She had taken a passionate prayer petition before God that morning. She told God she could not lose her mentor and closest friend and that she needed me. She reminded me that what I wanted to do more than anything is teach and preach God's word and see lives changed. She encouraged me to keep the vision before me. Don was so faithful and true to wait on me hand and foot. My grandson Addison did not miss a day visiting. He came for lunch every day for the first few weeks. Tears of love now flow easily. I am so thankful, especially for Don, my family, and my friends.

I was still awaiting final information from my physician but was concerned about what I might hear. At this point, my healthcare team consisted of my breast surgeon, plastic surgeon, and diagnostic radiologist. They met weekly with the East Texas Medical Center Tumor Board led by Dr. Fender, my breast surgeon. The Tumor Board is a group of physicians that includes surgeons, plastic surgeons, oncologists, radiation oncologists, diagnostic radiologists, and others. The team was waiting for input from the pathologist. They did not yet have information regarding the two receptor nodes that contained cancer cells. Detailed information regarding the nature of the cancer type in the cells would drive the recommendations for follow-up treatment - chemotherapy, radiation, chemotherapy medication? Oh my, all the possibilities sounded terrible. There were no good choices here. I just wanted this nightmare to end. I would receive their recommendations following the Tumor Board meeting discussion. And by the way, the chemotherapy would not start for at least a month following surgery. Hardly comforting at all.

August 11, 2016, I received the John Kilpatrick prayer handkerchief from my sister-in-law, Wanda. I placed it in one of the Home Depot painters apron pockets holding my drains on the right side. Holy Spirit said, 'The Father's Love.' That's what that anointed cloth represented in my life. I could feel the power of the Father's love.

In the beginning, my muscles were sore, and I was having a hard time lifting my arms to fix my hair. Don helped and made his first ponytail. I wrote in my journal, 'Yesterday is gone and has no binding power on your present or future.' Today is fleeting, a flash. God said I came to give you a future and a hope. Live today with a view toward tomorrow. Do you have the courage to bring forth treasures out of darkness? What can you do today to invest in the future God has shown you? Answer - 1. Well Within - a natural skincare product line God had birthed in me - speaking, educating, formulating, and promoting. 2. Writing. 3. Teaching and preaching God's word. 4. Invest in my family. I will not live by every word that proceeds out of the mouth of the doctors. I will live by every word that proceeds out of the mouth of God.

Seeing your purpose as God sees it gives you a future and a hope. Meditate on His word and His version of your future. It is full of life and possibility. He is my rock and my salvation. I don't trust anyone or anything other than Him. Rightly divide the word of truth. The truth that proceeds from the mouth of God. The word of God is active, alive, powerful, and sharper than any two-edged sword. Divides the soul and spirit issues of life. His words are life to all that find them and healing to all their flesh.

Chapter 14

UNCERTAINTY

August 12, 2016, I wrote,

My son, don't forget my instruction and keep my commandments carefully in mind. For they will add length to your days, years to your life, and abundant peace to you.
From Proverbs 3:1-26 ISV.

I started back to work in my home office. I began my weekly visits to Dr. Harrison for 'wound and scar watch' and filling of the chest expanders with saline. Ugh! After a few weeks, Dr. Harrison released me with a healthy scar, and my breast area was expanded as far as I wanted to grow. I was released to consult with the oncologist about chemotherapy, something I dreaded.

My internal war was raging. One day Jeremiah was telling God about the wretched, unfair circumstances of his life and his world as if God didn't already know. Jeremiah was a full-disclosure, no-holding-back man. He pleaded his case with God like a lawyer, telling Him that life is not fair. He told God that the people close to him were suffering. He explained that the wrong people were at ease and doing well. Those who were serving God only with their lips and not their hearts were fruitful. He explained that the situation was not fair. He said to God that he served Him with his whole heart and did everything He told him to do. Jeremiah described the misery he had endured. He asked God an eternal question - How long are You going to let this go on? Just wipe them out. That's the kind of justice I want. Because of these wicked men, the land is mourning, the grass and herbs are withering, the beasts and birds are dying. They are mocking like they are going to outlast me. Take this misery away. God replies,

> *If you have raced with men on foot and they have worn you out, how will you compete with horses? And if you stumble in a safe place, how will you manage in the thickets by the Jordan?*
> From Jeremiah 12:4,5 NIV.

In other words, Dorothy, you are not in Kansas anymore. Life is tough. There are lions, tigers, bears, and witches out there! Get up and be persistent in the battle to get from here to where I am taking you! It's a fight, but I'm taking you somewhere. Sometimes you can't see what I'm doing, but I'm working all things for your good, just the same. Sometimes you won't feel like getting up and moving forward. But if you don't look up, arise, and move forward, you will fall back and succumb. If you are going to die, die fighting. If you choose to live for a purpose, then fight for it.

Chapter 15

BECOMING THE WARRIOR PRINCESS

You know you've been assaulted at first, but you don't quite know what to make of the devastation. Damage assessment comes in bits and pieces. You cannot take it all in. Your mind tries to make order out of the ravages of war, but nothing is the same. The battle for my spirit, soul, and body was raging. I was learning to fight in a new way. And fight I did. The famous preacher, John Osteen, often encouraged people in the throes of battle by quoting these words by Edwin Markham,

> *Great it is to dream the dream while you're standing youth by the starry stream. But a greater thing is to fight life through and to say at the end, 'The Dream is True.'*

I would repeat these words over and over in my heart. They were life to me. These thoughts nurtured me as I stood to fight each moment, each day - a greater thing is to fight life through. These words grew in my heart, and so did my faith and determination to stay in the struggle. I was determined not to fall back and faint.

My precious Amanda and grandson River embedded the first warrior hologram on my heart. After learning of my diagnosis, Amanda sent me a handwritten card on June 15, 2016.

Jeanie, You know I'm not very good at phone calls, but I wanted to let you know how much you mean to me, and that I'm here for you anytime. The night Brian told me about your diagnosis, I went through so many emotions. I was angry and upset, thinking about how you finally got to work from home and enjoy the life you deserve. And then I thought, I know exactly how you would respond, "This is exactly the right time. God put me in this place in my life so that I could handle this while being home with Don." I then cried and cried, both for you and for all of us who have been so blessed to have had you in our lives. You taught me to think like that and to feel secure knowing that God has a plan for us and we are loved. I cried because I was so grateful to you, and because you are one of the very few people I've had in my life who I always know SEES me and LOVES me. And to have that from someone who I respect and love so deeply is one of the greatest gifts. I found peace in knowing who you are. You are so strong, yet loving. You are tough and a fighter, yet graceful. As I told River and described you in those terms, we then read your Facebook post where you used 'warrior.' We both exclaimed, "Mimi is Wonder Woman the Warrior Princess!" So I found this quote from Proverbs 31:25, which was perfect. You will beat this! I love you dearly! Love Amanda

Strength and honor are her clothing. She shall rejoice in time to come.
From Proverbs 31:25 NKJ

That image has burned in my heart ever since. Amanda and River gave me a word I could hold on to about a woman of valor. I began to see myself rising as Wonder Woman-Warrior Princess.

After all, I knew I was a new creation in Christ. God reminded me of the prophet and judge, Deborah. She was endowed with a prophetic gift - the ability to discern God's mind and purposes and declare it to others. She was a warrior princess. She was an innovative thinker and agitator. She was not afraid to stir up or incite riotous thought, public discussion with the view of producing a change. She awakened God's people with a determination to free themselves from their wretched bondage and degradation. She was a warrior who fought with words, warriors, and weapons. She was a woman with more courage than some men. God's people were being threatened. Genocide was the goal of the Canaanites. They were determined to kill all of God's people or take them into slavery. The threat was imminent. God's people were out armed and outmanned. They were outnumbered ten to one. Sisera, the leader of the Canaanites, had nine hundred iron chariots. That would be like having nine hundred of the best army tanks. Deborah was married to Lapidoth, but he was no help. She had a reluctant army commander, Barak. He said he would go into battle only if she went with him. Deborah was not afraid of the fight. God told her what was going to happen ahead of time. Because of that, she became a successful war strategist. She fought the battle on earth with God's strategy and weapons of war. This warrior knew God, and He gave His secret weapons-a woman from a neighboring clan and a tent peg! I saw myself as Wonder Woman and Deborah! I was becoming a Warrior Princess. I went to war with God's secret weapons.

Valor means the strength of mind or spirit that enables a person to encounter danger with firmness and personal bravery. I was learning to be that person of courage. Now, as I write this book, over three years later, I am a different person. I have authored and published my first book, *Mindful Meditation: 30 Days Uniting with the Heart of God*. I am not the same person. The battle will cost you all you've got, and then God deposits in you things you never imagined you could be. Don't be afraid of the process.

My son Tim reminded me of my new identity. My husband and I were driving on the interstate, trying to get to a football game to watch my granddaughter, Emma, cheer. We were pushing through a torrential rainstorm with strong winds and lightning. We could not see the highway in front of us. Sheets of rain beat down on us. I texted Tim and told him the weather was dangerous and getting worse. We were turning around to go back home. He called immediately and exclaimed, "Mom, where's your warrior spirit?" I laughed and reminded myself of who I was becoming. We pushed through.

Chapter 16

PATIENT PERSISTENCE THROUGH THREAT AND PAIN

The apostle Paul was the best at teaching our position in times of uncertainty. From the moment Paul encountered Christ on the road to Damascus, he lived, embraced, ran toward, did not shrink back from fearful situations. He was confident of his position in Christ, and nothing else mattered. He wanted others to have that same assurance.

> *I want you to know, dear ones, what has happened to me has not hindered but helped my ministry of preaching the gospel, causing it to expand and spread to many people.*
> From Philippians 1:12 TPT.

Every word Paul spoke was with certainty. He knew Jesus Christ brought the good news that could save your soul and so much more. Paul taught us that 'so much more.' I journaled that day, 'I live by every word that proceeds from the mouth of God - the proceeding, life-giving word of God. I submit myself under the mighty hand of God.' My Meditation, August 14, 2016:

Praise the Lord, all you nations. Extol Him, all you peoples. For great is His love toward us and the faithfulness of the Lord endures forever.
From Psalm 117:1,2. NIV

Praise the Lord. Lose your mind, your old way of thinking, so you can see what God wants you to see. Allow His thoughts to bubble to the top. Faith believes as real fact what is not revealed to the senses. If you'll step into this realm with Him and not look at the natural, you will see the supernatural. Walk in the things He has for you to walk in. He did not create the world from things you can see. He designed and built it with things that, at that time, were not visible.

Now back to the process. Being active was one of the best things I could do to recover and maintain good health. One Saturday, soon after the mastectomy, my daughter-in-law, Melissa, invited me to a Yoga class taught by her friend, Gina. Whew! That's when I realized the mastectomy had compromised all my upper body muscles. I set out on a mission to strengthen my arm, shoulder, and chest muscles. I had to be ready for opening deer season weekend, November 5th. Those deer rifles are heavy. I love to deer hunt and had not missed a deer yet, even though I had only been hunting a few years. I stayed focused on the goal of being able to lift and control my deer rifle. I gently exercised every day that I could. My son, Tim, taught me that just a little, purposeful activity and weight training could be as effective as a lot. I was persistent and consistent. I kept my eyes on the deer-hunting prize. We had shared many happy memories with family and friends at the deer lease. I wanted to be healthy and active again. My goal was to live life to the fullest.

Don and I had entered the cancer arena. For weeks I had been studying online through a group called The Truth About Cancer. My sister-in-law, Wanda, had introduced it to me a few weeks before my diagnosis. Now I was studying as if my life depended on it. I learned about alternative methods to diagnose and treat cancer. I learned about alternative treatment centers in the United States and around the world. I was not sure what my choice would be. Of course, my physicians recommended the usual route - cut it out, try to kill it with harmful chemicals, and burn it with radiation. I had already taken their first recommendation to cut it out. Now they were saying I needed to do more.

On September 8th, my first visit with the oncologist, Dr. Usrey, was quite unnerving. I was afraid. I regrouped on the inside. I knew that the opposing and most significant enemy of fear is love. I determined that day and every visit following that I would give love to each person I met. Love was a force greater than fear, and I was getting better at exercising my love, trust, and faith muscles. The first step of the oncology visit is always labs - blood draw. The blood lab waiting area was populated with people in various stages of cancer treatment. I got a glimpse of my future. I saw how courageous each one was, no matter what their current circumstance. I saw great grace on display in the middle of threat and danger. I eagerly grabbed courage from each one. Don and I easily engaged in conversation with all. Some of them eagerly shared their story.

After they drew what seemed to be gallons of blood, we waited to see the doctor. Dr. Usrey's nurse greeted us with a welcoming smile, weighed me, and took us to Dr. Usrey's office. The young doctor greeted us, looked at my blood test results, then started gushing with compliments about my blood. "Oh my, you have the blood of a 50-year-old woman!" That was quite a blessing since I had recently turned 69. I thought, at least I'm going into this battle with a strong body. But if I have a healthy body, how did I get cancer? That question still baffles me, and I continue to put together clues to unravel the mystery - stress, diet, genes, cosmetics, hair products, water? I am still on a quest to improve my health and educate others based on my learning.

Dr. Usrey began to discuss the pathology findings, the Tumor Board recommendations for treatment, and his counsel. I was somewhat reluctant to undergo any further treatment and asked lots of questions. What was the chemotherapy designed to do? Did I have any more cancer cells in my body?

He explained that I had two different breast cancers. The larger one was Stage 1 Invasive Ductal. The other was Pleomorphic Lobular Carcinoma. Two of the four sentinel lymph nodes they had mapped from the breast cancer tumors contained cancer cells. The breast that housed the cancerous tumors and the lymph nodes containing cancer had been surgically removed. The next recommended treatment was chemotherapy, a systematic treatment designed to destroy any cancer cells throughout my body. I learned that a patient could have micrometastases throughout the body that cannot be detected with any currently available tests. An effective systemic treatment is needed to cleanse the body of micrometastases to improve a patient's duration of survival and potential for cure. That is the oncologist's reasoning for adjuvant therapy. Adjuvant means 'to help.' Adjuvant therapy is additional therapy given after surgery when all detectable disease has been removed, but there remains a statistical risk of relapse due to undetected disease. I pressed Dr. Usrey with many questions and asked about healthier options. How did he know I needed this? He rared back in his chair and said, "For all we know, you may not have any cancer cells in your body at all." I felt uneasy as if this was one big crapshoot.

So now the ball was back in my court. We were discussing what may or may not be in my body and survival rate. Oh my! How did we get here? The cancer world is an ever-unfolding mystery full of what-ifs and statistical probability. Dr. Usrey's recommendation for me was chemotherapy with Adriamycin, dose-dense treatment, meaning every two weeks, for eight weeks followed by Cytoxin, dose-dense, for eight weeks. Dr. Usrey explained that most oncologists on the Tumor Board had recommended another chemotherapy drug rather than Adriamycin. Adriamycin is commonly known as 'the red devil' because the side effects are so harsh. Side effects include neuropathy, low blood count, nausea, hair loss. The risks can also include the potential to damage the heart, causing it not to pump as well. It damages the cancer DNA and can damage your own DNA (less than 1% chance), resulting in new cancer like leukemia down the road. But Dr. Usrey believed it to be the most effective treatment for me and thought my body could take it. To verify that this recommended course of treatment was the most effective, I consulted a physician and friend, Dr. Melody Smith, Hematologic Oncologist. She researches at Memorial Sloan Kettering Cancer Center. After I explained my diagnosis to Melody and Dr. Usrey's proposed course of treatment, she confirmed that Dr. Usrey's recommendations were precisely the treatment course recommended for my condition by physicians at their hospital. I still vacillated between natural, alternative therapy, and chemotherapy. I discussed it with my husband and family. All were in agreement to follow the doctor's orders. They wanted to see me live a long life and thought this was the best way. I scheduled my first chemotherapy treatment for Wednesday, September 14th.

I must interject here that you have the right and privilege to choose your personal pathway of health and healing. Do your research. Ask lots of questions. Keep a journal. Prepare your questions before the visit with your physician. Take your time. Your doctor may be in a hurry, but you are not. You want to get this right. Write the answers to your questions in your journal. Trust me, you will not recall all that your doctor says. It's a new world, a new reality. You are learning to make this your world where you are in control and making informed decisions. Take someone with you to your physician visits - your healthcare partner. My husband faithfully went with me to each visit. Your healthcare partner will remember things you don't and may have a more objective perspective. Dr. Usrey later lovingly laughed and said, "Oh, you are the person that came in with a list of questions. I always wondered when you would get to the last one." At each visit, he paused and set aside as much time as it took to answer each of my questions based on recent research. As a patient, I felt honored, respected, and supported.

Before I could begin chemotherapy, I was scheduled for an echocardiogram to look at my heart function. The oncology team would stop the Adriamycin treatment if my heart showed signs of trouble. I was also scheduled to have a PICC (Peripherally Inserted Central Catheter) line inserted to deliver the chemotherapy. It's like a long IV line that stays in your body for the duration of chemotherapy treatment. It's a long, thin, hollow tube inserted into a vein in the upper arm around the elbow and ends in a larger vein in the chest wall near the heart. It was an annoying, uncomfortable, but necessary part of me for over four months. I could not get the insertion site wet, so showers were a challenge. Don and I developed creative ways to keep it dry.

On September 13, 2016, I spoke with Janne Swearengen, my great uncle Larry's wife. She had been diagnosed with breast cancer a few years back and had undergone a lumpectomy with no chemotherapy recommended. She had taken hormone-blocking medication following the lumpectomy. She soon went rogue and stopped taking it when the side-effects she encountered were not worth the benefit of the medicine. She knew I was going for my first chemotherapy treatment the next day. She said, "I will have you in my thoughts tomorrow as the new regimen begins. Are you keeping a journal of your thoughts, reactions, questions, and emotions?" I thought, "Geez! My thoughts are wild, random, crazy. Like I am rocking and jerking on a turbulent ride at an amusement park. I am walking toward something I don't want to do, but I must. I'm walking in blind and afraid, knowing it will be rough but believing everything will be alright in the end. I'm sitting on the front row of a movie theater at a horror flick's opening scene. It's almost real. I watch it with one eye closed. It's not me in the scene, but I experience all the emotions. In the end, I come out unscathed and greatly relieved." I knew Janne was right, and I became more faithful, making regular entries in my journal, writing the raw truth.

One of the greatest weapons of the enemy is fear - fear of the unknown, fear of exposing your vulnerability in front of others, fear of sickness, fear of death. But to Christians, sometimes the most significant concern is, "What if I totally trust God, and I am disappointed?" All of us have been disappointed, and it hurts deeply. Sometimes we lose hope. We lose our ability to trust God. But what if we believe Him with all that is within us, and He blesses us far above what we can imagine or think? I don't know about you, but I want to use my imagination to see what God has in store for me. Trust in the Lord with your whole heart (not half), and don't try to understand everything. Look for Him to direct all your ways. He will take over and direct your path. (My version of Proverbs 3:5) Faith begins when we get information from God. God informed Noah of things that had never been seen - rain and flooding. I want to see the unseen and reach into the unknown. God will not disappoint! He wants me to know the mysteries of His kingdom.

I was walking through the valley of the shadow where the blanket of darkness lowered over me. It's a familiar human excursion. Walking through the canyon with a heart full of threatening haze, we feel desperate. You've had faith, but now it's waning. Tempted to anticipate a bright future, you fall back into gloom. Disappointment might kill you. You have believed before but lost all hope when things did not work out. If you expect too much, disapointment could turn your heart to stone. You can't even admit to yourself, but you might be disappointed with God. The waters are murky and foreboding. You've got your eyes closed because you will die of fright if you see what's there. The cloaked specters are too large and loud. With His ark of security, the Lord will carry you through on top of His rushing river of truth. His light will come, and the shifting shadows will flee away. He will take away your sorrow and your disappointment with God. He will carry you through and renew your faith. You will flow through the valley on the river of God.

I felt like a staggering boxer, answering each punch with a counterpunch. Just the thought of chemotherapy made me sick and scared. I had taken such good care of my body, and now I was to follow a treatment protocol (such cold words) just because research said it might work. Our oncologist was kind. He always looked for ways to comfort me. But I was afraid. I began to cry out for life - His life in my body. I yearned for His resurrection life in each cell of my body. I was in the fight of my life. Deep calls to deep! I called from deep inside to touch the True and Living God. I knew what God's word said about me.

The Law of the Spirit of Life in Christ Jesus made me free from the Law of Sin and Death.
From Romans 8:2 NKJ.

I embraced the Law of the Spirit of Life in Christ Jesus and all its potential power.

Chapter 17

CHEMOTHERAPY CHAMPION

My first chemotherapy treatment was Wednesday, September 14, 2016. I had not positively embraced this little visit at all. On the day of my first treatment, I wrote, 'You are entering the arena, and you are afraid. With the strength of God, just do it afraid with your eyes wide open. Don't flinch. Don't shrink back.' I had taken such good care of my body. I reached up to God for re-visioning. God gave me a picture of liquid honey flowing from heaven, flowing down over my head and all over me. God's warm and nourishing honey-love. Life is not always fair. Live it out with God and extraordinary grace.

I signed multiple consent forms and was given instructions before treatment began. The oncologist had written a wig prescription. The prescription read, 'Cranial prosthesis for chemo-induced alopecia. Dx C50.411 - malignant neo R female breast.' Oh my! I could hardly take it in! It felt like the blows just kept on coming! I was also given access to their resource room. I found books written to support people going through cancer treatment and hats to cover bare heads. The books were available for checkout. I was looking for anything to help me understand all this, but all I wanted to read was someone else's story, told from the heart. All the books I found were educational and stale. No author was there to reveal the real story from a human perspective. Later I was to find Deanna Favre's book online. She wrote *Don't Bet Against Me*. It's her personal story of life from breast cancer diagnosis to the founding of the Deanna Favre Hope Foundation. Her crisis carried her to a new purpose. Her foundation supports breast cancer education, women's breast imaging, and diagnostic services for all women, including those who are medically underserved. I bought the Kindle version and read it at bedtime, in the dark, through my tears.

The nurse gave me several prescription medications to prevent nausea and told me how to take them. The nurse explained that hair-loss would begin two to three weeks following day one of chemotherapy. I was dazed. Baldness would begin two weeks from today. My hair would start growing back about one month following my last chemotherapy treatment. I was told I would lose my appetite but to eat anyway - high protein shakes, etc. I might experience heart function changes, chest pain, heart flutter, heart racing. My mouth might get sore. In that case, I was to rinse with one teaspoon baking soda and salt throughout the day. I might experience bladder functioning changes and bleeding. I was to drink eight to ten glasses of water each day and empty my bladder frequently. My immune system would begin to be compromised. Within 10-14 days, I might experience decreased white blood count, decreased red blood cells, and reduced platelet counts. I was to wash my hands often and stay away from sick people. The nurse patched a small, rectangular box on my arm called Neulasta. It worked as a bone marrow stimulant and white blood cell booster. She set the timer to deploy 24 hours following the chemotherapy treatment. It would begin to tick a few seconds before it began, giving me an injection in the arm. Its purpose was to help my body produce white blood cells, reducing my risk of infection during intense chemotherapy. I grew to hate it, but it became my best friend. Neulasta came with its own side-effects, but I never got an infection during the entire course of my chemotherapy treatment. The nurse educated me on all potential side-effects from chemotherapy and Neulasta. I was to call the doctor if my temperature went above 100 degrees.

The saline bag mixed with my chemotherapy prescription was connected to the PICC line in my arm. First, I received an infusion of Adriamycin (the red devil AKA Doxorubicin) for five to ten minutes, followed by a Cytoxan drip for 30 minutes. I had learned that chemotherapy could cause cancer. I saw the warning on the chemotherapy drip bag. Hard to believe, but it is true. I saw it with my own eyes. There were some other things dripped into me that day, including medication to decrease inflammation. My total treatment time was about two hours. I had taken books, my Kindle, and crocheting to keep me occupied. I would take them out of my bag, but I rarely needed them. I always found people to talk to who were receiving chemotherapy. I enjoyed chatting with patients and their families. I was always encouraged by their stories. I also found ways to support them. Don brought me lunch from a local restaurant to eat during treatment. I knew it was essential to maintain a healthy diet. I did my best throughout treatment to give my body the nutrients needed to promote every cell's health. Following my first chemotherapy infusion, I went home and back to work in my home office. I felt a little different that day, but I was not falling apart. My friend Karen called me that night. We talked about the battle. She is a great Christian and continuously called to support me. She challenged me with, "Sometimes you lose the game before you play it by the thoughts you choose to entertain." I was determined to play this game and win-win the battle in my mind and my body.

By Friday evening, September 16, 2016, chemotherapy side effects had set in. I found that this was to be the pattern throughout my course of treatment with Adriamycin. I would receive chemotherapy on Wednesday, and then full side effects would begin Friday evening. My symptoms were shortness of breath, pain around the PICC line insertion site, tenderness and swelling around my shoulders, nausea, heart racing, overall weakness, and blurred vision. I was tired throughout the weekend. About all I could do was lay around. Don took great care of me, preparing healthy food, and making sure I rested. We watched a lot of college football and were thankful to have each other. I stopped taking my nausea medication on Saturday because it was not helping. The nausea was not that bad. The nausea meds were creating the blurred vision and contributing to exhaustion. The heart-racing created anxiety, but it was not constant. I checked it all out with my physician. It was all part of the chemotherapy side effects.

Chapter 18

LIVING LIFE ON DIFFERENT LEVELS

On Monday, September 19, 2016, it was time to go back to work. I was still tired, and any kind of activity was exhausting. But work was a diversion. It kept me from dwelling on the way I was feeling. Because I was working from home, it was easy to get up in the morning, get my coffee, go to my home office, and start my day. I did not have to get up and get dressed. That alone would have been exhausting. I wrote in my journal that day as God spoke to my heart:

This is a marathon and not a sprint. I have prepared you and am preparing you with signs, wisdom, wonders, and grace to stand and win this race. When I said, 'This is my body broken for you,' I meant it's broken, so you don't have to endure any of the same unless there is an overflowing payoff for My kingdom. As you seek me in your suffering, I am creating a future and a hope for you with great benefits.

God gave me heavenly vision and provision. On the evening of Wednesday, September 21, 2016, I was crying out to God. I felt terrible. My hair was beginning to fall out. And I had gotten it trimmed that day, pixie style. God showed me a vision of a horse and rider. TRUST, written like a banner across the image, jumped to the front. Immediately my understander tried to figure out whether I was the horse or the rider. I tried out several scenarios in my mind - me as the horse and God as a rider or me as rider and God as the horse. Try as I may, my understander could not settle on the truth. Finally, I asked God, "Who is the horse, and who is the rider?" He immediately said, "We're one!" We are one. No separation. One. TRUST. My friend Karen knows so much about riding and training horses. She explained that when riding your horse, you want cadence. It takes trust and the right cues for a horse and rider to enter into confidence and rhythm. Cadence is the beat, time, or measure of rhythmical motion or activity - tempo. Trust is developed over time as the horse and rider learn to work together in harmony. The horse and rider become as one. I have grown to trust what Paul the Apostle said.

Christ in me, the hope of glory.
From Colossians 1: 27 NKJV.

As I followed the yellow brick road of promise, I was walking and working it out. There were giants I had to face. Fear was looming large like dark, low-lying clouds with the promise of brewing storms. The Bible lessons I had once learned, and even taught, were now empty to me. The chemotherapy I was taking was trying to pull me down a dark hole - spirit, soul, and body. I verified with my friend Veronica, a nurse, who had gone through the same treatment with Adriamycin, the red devil. She agreed. It tried to take all of her, within and without, sucking her down the sinkhole. I felt like I was circling the drain. I had to face the giants with God leading me. Once again, I was face-to-face with fear.

I was on the firing line with fear laying down the gauntlet. The burgeoning civil war was rumbling. Fear is chilling - cold as ice. If you let fear have his way, he will start with a cold stab to your heart. He is relentless. He's not satisfied with your heart. He flows throughout your body, coursing through each artery and vein. Your skin begins to crawl with an expectancy of the worst. Fear whispers real loud that he is commanding the circumstances of your life, and you can't do anything about it. He is an artist who paints pictures that haunt and linger. He begins to direct the theater in your mind like a talented producer. At the onset of his production, you think these thoughts are your own because they're hissing in your head. You can see your future unfold day-by-day, moment-by-moment, with disappointment, pain, and sorrow. You see yourself drowning in the ocean with no life preserver. You move forward quickly to your end - your funeral. You have lost life and are no longer among the living - everyone you love and all who love you can't cross over.

But God! There is a battle to be fought and territory to be taken. David once spoke,

Whenever I was in distress, you enlarged me.
From Psalm 4:1 TPT.

I counted on the promise knowing I could fight the good fight of faith and that God was in control of each skirmish, every battle, and the finale. As I stood up trusting God, I grew heads above the enemy. When I was out of control, I could trust God to be in control. I threw myself at His feet. He lifted me into His arms and held me tight. Fear is His enemy, too. He enjoys dissipating fear's spell, rendering him powerless.

My courage was emerging. Courage cannot exist without an ominous threat when there is a real possibility of damage or danger. Fear wants to immobilize you and bully you into confusion and retreat. You can turn your fear into fuel to fight. You must move forward in the face of fear. Do it afraid. Take a deep breath and move forward. You will be met with new ground, a place to stand and withstand the enemy. I was facing a new giant, and like David facing Goliath, I stepped out to win. There are many contradictions in life. Bad things happen to good people. The contradictions of life cause dissonance in your system. Everything is topsy-turvy. The way you thought it would be is not. Things don't make sense. You are being defined by how you respond to unpredictable, perplexing events. You are becoming a fearless warrior.

I was taking a chemical sentimental journey. Chemotherapy was stripping me of my human-made defense system. I was becoming more emotionally sensitive. I was experiencing life differently, like an artist with a palette full of new, full-spectrum colors. My grandmother Elizabeth was like that - tears came to her eyes very quickly. She had endured hard times and had maintained her stability. She was soft yet durable. Difficulties had dug out a well full of feelings. She had a comforting bosom with bountiful love and acceptance. She cared deeply about others, and it showed in so many ways. As my father had said to me many years ago on a long drive from Albuquerque to Colorado Springs, "Jean, my emotions are sensitive and full range like a piano that plays on all eighty-eight keys."

Who are you when everything has been stripped away? Nothing powerful ever comes uncontested. Struggle is strengthening. Suffering has value. Nobody gets through this world without it. You learn lessons by persisting through hardship. In the end the pain of suffering is gone but the lessons learned never leave you.

Chapter 19

Hair Today Gone Tomorrow

On September 28, 2016, I had my second chemotherapy treatment. Hair loss was to start two to three weeks following the first dose of chemotherapy. Kelly Mosley had styled my hair for years. She had faithfully come to my home following the mastectomy to cut and color my hair. I wanted to look my best even though I was now breastless. Kelly had helped others through the same breast cancer journey. She was on standby to help me in any way possible. I loved my hair. It had covered my head and framed my face since I was a child. It had been permed, colored, cut, washed, dried, curled, and sprayed for decades. I had spent thousands of hours and lots of money over my lifetime to have pretty hair. It was a part of me. Following my first chemotherapy treatment, I vigilantly studied my hair daily. I washed it, curled it, shaped it, and sprayed it. I was not losing any hair. I thought maybe I was going to be the exception. This chemotherapy was not going to affect me the way it had others. But like clockwork, two weeks following my first treatment, I started noticing more hair on my pillow. It looked like a fluffy cat had been laying on it.

I can't explain the grief that comes with losing your hair. It was coming out fast as fairy dust off Tinkerbell's toes. I had to comb it outside, with strands following the wind. I needed to sleep on a cat bed. I discussed my hair loss details with my son, Brian. He advised, "Mom, you don't want to look like the zombie apocalypse!" That day I wrote, 'My God is my glory. He lifts my head. I love Him so. Tonight, I will have to look up zombie apocalypse to see what Brian means.' My cosmetologist and friend, Kelly, had suggested cutting it short. On September 29, 2016, Don took me to get a pixie cut. We laughed and cried as the scissors sang close to my scalp. Kelly gave me some beautiful flowers.

My vanity and vulnerability surfaced. Losing my hair was very hard. This new Peter Pan hairstyle was not me, but this was now my reality. I had been dealt a bad hand and had to play it. Too late to ask for a re-deal. That was a tough day, but at least my hair was styled. Then I began losing hair at a faster rate. Combing my hair outside was the new norm. I was shedding like a furry critter in the midsummer heat. My sorrow was mounting, but I didn't let it show. I was holding on to God with all the strength I had. I did not know He was holding on to me, carrying me to safety like a mother cat takes her babies to a secure hiding place. But my hair continued to fall out. The pillow I slept on was covered with hair every morning. When I would comb my hair in the house, it would come off in the wide-toothed comb. I went outside to fix my hair. I watched it fall to the ground. My happy thought was that a bird or squirrel could use it as part of their building materials for a warm nest. Hair was everywhere but on my head - on my clothes, in the shower, in my bed. I just need to get rid of it. Shave it off.

This chemo-triggered molting gathered momentum. I got brave enough to discuss it with Don. One morning I came inside after combing my hair, watching strands whirl through the atmosphere. My husband said, "Why don't we go ahead and cut it all off." I laughed and agreed. We would cut it after work that evening in the backyard. On the evening of October 3, 2016, after I finished work, we gathered what we needed - a chair, a sheet to wrap around me, scissors, and shears. Oh my! Were we doing this? Shears?

Don said we might as well shave it all off. I wanted to say 'no,' but I knew he was right. We positioned the chair in the backyard in the grass. It was an occasion we will never forget. I cried, but Don made me laugh through my tears. We both smiled as hair drifted everywhere. The deed was done. Now it was time to live life with grace and a bald head.

Good grief, Charley Brown, this is hard. It had now been two days since the shaving. I had only looked in the mirror once since Don exposed my naked head. It's now two mornings later. Vanity! Identity! I've always enjoyed being Jean. I had recognized that I had the basics of an attractive person. I could put on a little makeup, fix my hair, and put on cute clothes to enhance what I had. But now, it was hard to look in the mirror without hair covering. So I wore a hat or scarf to cover my hairlessness. It's hard to say the word 'bald.' I also needed to keep my head warm.

Even though the oncologist and nurse had warned that hair loss would happen, I was shocked and heart-sick. I just thought I would be the exception and that it would not happen to me. But then again, I never thought I would be diagnosed with cancer either. I was embarrassed too. I did not want Don to see me without hair. Like all women, I always wanted to feel attractive. I especially wanted to be pretty for him. But it was hard to hide. I kept something on my head all the time. My head was cold, my scalp was tender, and I loved having a crown of glory, even if I designed it myself. Each time I would see anything in my home associated with hair, sorrow would overtake me. I hid everything associated with fixing hair - combs, brushes, hairdryer, flat iron, bobby pins, hair spray, etc. You would be surprised how many items you use just to support beautiful hair. When we went to the deer lease, I opened a cabinet in our fifth wheel and exposed more objects associated with haircare. I hid them all. A friend who went through the same journey told me she threw everything away associated with hair so she would not be reminded of hair loss, although when you look in the mirror, it's hard to miss. Another friend told me that hair loss was the most disturbing side-effect for her dad when he went through chemotherapy. Although I pushed back all reminders that I did not have hair, I needed to transition to the new me. My crown of glory for the next few months would be beautiful scarves, hats, and wigs. I had to accept it and be content. One study followed a group of women who experienced hair loss after chemotherapy and found four reactions common to most of the group: not prepared, shocked, embarrassed, and feeling a loss of a sense of self. For some women, hair loss was more psychologically painful than the loss of a breast through cancer.

For me, head covering was essential. Before the chemotherapy treatments began, we had been advised to purchase a wig. The advice was to select a hairpiece similar to my current hair color and style. The wig selection event was very emotional for me - surreal. Was this happening to me? As usual, Don made it fun. We went shopping for a wig that was cute and close to my hair color. At that time, I still had hair. As I looked around at all the head-covering options, I was solemn, still, and cold as steel on the inside. On the outside, I smiled and deflected my anxious thoughts to hold back the tears. Don worked so hard to encourage me. The shop-keeper talked to me with the voice of experience while I looked around. She shared other breast cancer shoppers' experiences.

We selected a wig that was cute and synthetic. After becoming hairless, I wore it a few times, but it was uncomfortable. My scalp was sensitive. My friend Karen gave me a beautiful blonde wig made of real human hair. I wore it and felt glamorous. I bought some hats that made me happy. They were fun to wear around the house. My head was cold when it was not covered. Besides, I wanted to celebrate life in little ways. I wore them with style. I began to develop my unique signature head-dresses - taking scarves and crafting fashionable turbans and head wraps. My granddaughter, Emma, and daughter-in-law, Melissa, helped me with one creative style while watching a football game on a Saturday. I had so much fun and got so many compliments. I was learning to enjoy what life had dealt and be me, unapologetically. Flaunting my new headpieces, I laughed and told everyone I wanted some tarot cards and a crystal ball for Christmas because

I was going to become a fortune-teller. That's not far from the truth. I do have some prophetic giftings.

An Interview with My Cosmetologist, Kelly Mosley

Me: What thoughts do people who are losing or have lost their hair express to you?

Kelly: Shock. No one can prepare you for the emotions you will go through when it happens. You've always seen yourself with hair on your head. You may have hairless baby pictures, but that's different. Hair is part of your personality, your identity. It's not vain or anything. Hair is an attachment to your body and makes you who you are. No one can be prepared for how fast hair loss can happen and how quickly the process unfolds. You may be devastated. In a couple of days, you can go from a full head of hair to nothing. It's a loss that must be grieved. At the same time, you are facing other health issues associated with your treatment. You are also coming to terms with your diagnosis. No one can prepare you for all of that. You are exposed, and everybody that sees you knows what you are going through. You may not be ready to talk about it at the time. There is no way to hide it. Yes, you can wear a wig or a hat. You can be bold and go without a head covering. But it's something you can't guard against emotionally or physically. It's just out there.

Me: Why do you think it's so hard for people to lose their hair?

Kelly: It's like a blanket. It's a comforter. It's our shield. It helps keep us warm. It's a part of us. Baldness bothers everybody, whether it's hereditary or alopecia areata or the result of chemotherapy treatments. At least with chemotherapy, you know your hair is going to come back. With some other types of hair loss, it never grows back.

Me: So you have had male customers who have dealt with hair loss?

Kelly: Even the bald people may be embarrassed that they have to get their hair cut and styled to deal with baldness.

Me: What words of encouragement would you give to someone who is losing or has lost their hair?

Kelly: Embrace it. Know that you are not alone. If your hair loss is due to chemotherapy treatments, just know that your hair will come back. One of my prayers is, Lord, you know every hair on my head. They are all numbered. (From the words of Jesus, Luke 12:7) If you see every hair that I'm losing, please put them all back when I'm through.

Me: What else would you like to say to our readers?

Kelly: Get in a support group. Talk to others who have been through it. We must encourage one another. You don't know what it's like until you have gone through it. Nobody can understand until it happens to them.

Caring comfort often came well-timed. During this hairless season, my daughter-in-law Melissa came by to visit while Don and I were away from the house. She slipped into my home office and penned a sweet note, "Love you, Jean Elizabeth. You are beautiful and treasured beyond your beauty!" What a blessing that tender thought brought. That message is still posted above my desk. It's a daily reminder that true beauty is who you are and not what you look like.

Chapter 20

SHOW ME YOUR GLORY

On October 4, 2016, I wrote: I am being enlarged. I am stretched like a rubber band. My earthly glory is fading.

You, oh Lord, are a shield around me. You are my glory and the one who holds my head high.
From Psalm 3:3 NLT.

Therefore we do not lose heart. Though outwardly we are wasting away, yet inwardly we are being renewed day by day.
From 2 Corinthians 4:16 NIV.

Those who trust in the Lord will find new strength. They will soar high on wings like eagles. They will run and not grow weary. They will walk and not faint.
From Isaiah 40:31 NLT.

I wait upon the Lord, and He renews my strength so I can mount up like wings of eagles. I want to fly. I want to soar.

Oh my, Don called, and the kids are coming for dinner. How much do you believe in God's word? Let His glory rise. My earthly glory is fading. I was ready. Lord, you are my glory, my covering. Their visit is such a blessing.

A faithful friend covers all. On October 4, 2016, my husband told our friend Don Fisher about the 'hair saga.' Don told my husband, "I've been thinking about that, and I've got a lot of caps. I'm going to go through them and give her some." That touched me deep in my soul and spirit. I felt the love and compassion flowing from a friend! I love you for that, Don Fisher.

I am enjoying my sensitivity to God, to man, and to events. The whole world looks different to me as I experience great need with His beauty and grace right in its midst.

I became sensitive to other-worldliness. On October 6, 2016, I began to write: Sometimes, I am aware of two realms at one time. The other night I was lying in bed. Out of the corner of my eye, I saw my dad and others entering the room. It was as if my dad was trying to walk incognito. He was facing forward and did not look my way. He had a gray mustache. I guess he's got work to do here.

Today I felt my father standing behind me while I was working at my desk. He placed his hand on my shoulder and held it as if he was trying to brace me, stabilize me, and get me to hold my shoulders back. The whole room was flooded with angels. I sat up straight and smiled with the peace of God, knowing His grace and His embrace was here.

On October 7, 2016, I wrote: I am under His tutelage. God challenged me to read the New Testament and the Book of Psalms with my current-circumstance glasses on. Go to Hebrews. Devour it. Let it be your necessary food. Crack the codes.

> *Blessed is the man that does not walk in the counsel of the ungodly, nor stands in the path of sinners, nor sits in the seat of the scornful. Let your delight be in the law of the Lord and meditate in it day and night. You will*

be like a tree firmly planted by streams, rivers of water. The tree yields its fruit in its season. Your leaf, foliage, does not wither. All that you do shall prosper.
From Psalm 1:1-3 NKJV.

Fruit trees must be pruned during a specific season to produce more and better fruit. Pruning includes cutting and removing of selected parts of a fruit tree. Branches are cut back, and smaller limbs may be removed entirely. It may also involve eliminating young shoots, buds, and leaves. Many years ago, we had a peach tree that bore many small peaches each year. I began to study how to care for peach trees. The recommendation was to cut entire branches back severely. Ouch! It just didn't seem right, but that winter, I did it anyway. The following summer, we had plenty of blooms that gave way to clusters of small, green peaches (buds). Then I read that to have larger peaches, I should pick some of the green fruit off the groups of emerging pods. Where there was a cluster of three, I removed two small, green peaches. Sure enough, the peaches grew into large, sweet fruit.

The cutting back and early pruning did not seem right to me. And the tree seemed happy doing what it wanted to do - growing willy-nilly, without direction, haphazardly. I know the pruning hurt. But the pain gave way to better fruit. It took faith to believe that painful pruning would bring a better product. Pruning looked like it might bring death. But I found that pain with patience yielded better peaches. Life and circumstances try the hearts of men. Some seasons are painful. We don't understand what is happening to us or why. Some seasons we feel dormant and dry. We are chilled to the bone with fear of what might happen next. I was learning to trust God in the winter of my soul. He was pruning back what needed to go, so God's life could emerge in all its glory.

On October 8, 2016, I wrote:

Even in times of trouble. I have a joyful confidence, knowing that my pressures will develop in me patient endurance. And the patient endurance will refine my character, and proven character leads me back to hope. And

this hope is not a disappointing fantasy, because I can now experience the endless love of God cascading into my heart through the Holy Spirit who lives in me!
From Romans 5:3-5 TPT.

My friends, consider yourself fortunate when all kinds of trials come your way. For you know that when your faith succeeds in facing such trials, the result is the ability to endure. Make sure that your endurance carries you all the way without failing so that you may be perfect and complete lacking nothing. But if any of you lack wisdom, you should pray to God, who will give it to you. For God gives generously and graciously to all.
From James 1:2-5 GNT.

Sometimes the winds of life are contrary. Storms are brewing and the foamy, tempest-tossed waves are crashing over your head. Trust Him to navigate you safely to shore.

October 9, 2016, I rested in:

He took note of their distress when he heard their cry. For their sake He remembered His covenant, and out of His great love He relented. He caused all who held them captive to show them mercy.
From Psalm 106:44-46 NIV.

Chapter 21

LITTLE LOST LAMB

Chemotherapy induced brain fog was closing in, affecting my mental visibility. My skull was soaked with damp cotton. I had concentration and memory problems. Inability to find words mid-sentence was unsettling to me as a speech-language pathologist. I was determined to navigate my aircraft safely through the murky haze. Auto-pilot took over as I grew to rely on my instrument panel and flew in under the radar of the enemy.

On October 16, 2016, I wrote: All day yesterday Holy Spirit kept saying 'verse 176'. I knew the Bible inside out but could not figure out where that could be until last night. Suddenly the longest chapter in the Bible, Psalm 119, popped into my head. Searching, I thought surely that chapter does not have 176 verses. But there it was, the very last verse.

I have strayed like a lost sheep. Seek your servant. For I have not forgotten your commandments.
From Psalm 119:176 NIV.

Look for me, God, for I am lost in a place I do not want to be - a land of discomfort and dread. I long to be well again. I want to be healthy and happy, joyfully leading others. You are leading me in Your paths of righteousness for Your name's sake, Jesus. You have plans to give me a future and a hope. I know that wherever I am, you are with me. Seek me, find me, lead me, teach me.

The Good Shepherd is pulling me off the rocky precipice through the brambles. I'm drawn through this space of grace, hooked by the crook of His rod. When I'm lost, He searches for me, using the staff to part harsh terrain. An insistent poke shouts, "Don't wander off the path." When life-circumstances thrust me to threatening territory, He never stops searching. He defends me against the attacks of my predators. His rod and His staff comfort me. Moses climbed up the mountain through much darkness and uncertainty to get to God. I am overshadowed by darkness and doom, but God is in the darkness, directing me to an undisclosed destination.

The Lord has said that He would dwell in thick darkness.
From 1 Kings 8:12 ESV.

In times of alarm and dread, God plays show and tell. He reveals things unspeakable and full of glory, not yet seen or heard. The darkness is thick. You don't know where you are going. Listen in the dark. The enemy is looming large, but God's still small voice speaks volumes of comfort, wisdom, and guidance. Listen and look. Don't close your eyes in fear. He wants to show you things. Listen and look. Write what you see and hear. Later those words will be food to your starved soul.

Sheep are prey animals. A prey animal is one that is sought, captured, and eaten by a predator. The instinct to play 'follow the leader' is hardwired into the sheep's brain. They don't have to think about it. They stick close to the sheep in front of them. The paths they walk are not straight. They walk winding trails so they can see behind them, first with one eye then the other. They can watch for threats. Survival instincts cause them to flock together to avoid predators. They become highly agitated if they are separated from the group. When threatened by a predator, sheep flee, and in doing so, sometimes get lost. Sheep are very social animals. In a grazing situation, they need to see other sheep. During the cancer journey, I sometimes felt lost and vulnerable. Some of the cells in my body were out of control and wanted to lead me to death. The traditional cancer treatments were killing rogue cells and damaging some of my healthy cells. A battle was going on in my body and soul. I felt out of control. But the Good Shepherd was leading me through the valley of the shadow of death. The threatening, thick darkness was all around. But He was leading me the whole way. I fought to hear His voice amid the raging reality of death. My body and soul were under siege. He led me and fed me through the valley.

Faithful friends flock together. On October 6, 2016, I wrote: One of my most loyal friends in this fight was Karen Vestal. She loves me so much and walked beside me all the way. The feelings of my infirmities genuinely touched her. She called almost daily. When I was not able to answer, she left long, encouraging voicemails. When we talked, our conversations were synergistic and about how God was working in our lives. Each time we talked, God spoke something great 'among us.' She always admonished me to write about my experience. She knew God's grace is more extraordinary in hard times and that He was doing great things. She wanted to capture God's grace as it was happening for herself and others. Last night she called and left a voicemail saying, "Look up Habakkuk 2:2 and tell me what it means to you." It says,

Write the vision and make it plain on tablets, that he may run who reads it. From Habakkuk 2:2 NKJ

Karen said she wants my words ready when she or others need it. I love her so. She is such an inspiration to me and many others.

Sheep need to see other sheep. October 22, 2016, a visit from our faithful friends, Karen and Hubert Vestal, was just what the doctor ordered. Even when you don't feel as good as you would like, dress up and do life as though everything is fine. It was a beautiful, sunny fall day. Tim and his family came over to visit too. Karen and I shared so many God-thoughts. We believed God was preparing us for something. The meek shall inherit the earth. The gentleness of David made him great, but he was also a great warrior. David learned leadership by being a shepherd. He witnessed poor leadership when watching his father, Jessie, who was blinded by favoritism. He could not see the God-given DNA in his youngest son, David. David also experienced poor leadership with Saul. Saul only knew God with his head and lips. He did not know Him with his heart. His selfish ambition muddled his mind. He was centered on maintaining his own position of power. He was fearful and jealous of any rivals. Saul was ruled by his senses. He became harsh, and his weakness led to delusion and self-destruction. I want to be like David, a gentle yet brave warrior.

Chapter 22

LIVE LIFE LARGE IN THE MIDST OF THE STORM

You are in God's boot camp. Give what you don't have. Plant seeds in others out of the depths of your need. It will force you to give out of God and His resources. Get out of yourself and allow God to provide you with the grace to enjoy and give to others. God is a life-creator and a life-producer. He can create where a seed has not yet been planted if you give Him a place to grow His grace in your heart. Enjoy. Go and do likewise. We are creative beings just like our Father God. Give yourself space, His space, see what is unseen, and hear what is unheard. Say what you see and hear. He is your loving heavenly Father, and He cares for you. He is for you. Surrender. Don't be afraid of unveiling your silent, hidden potential. Watch what He does. See it, hear it, say it, do it when He whispers, 'Go.'

In each season, life brings surprises, challenges, and opportunities. We don't always know what is going to happen next. Cancer was a huge surprise to me. I was knocked down, but I did not stay down. I dug deeper than I had ever before while tightening my grip on truth and sanity. God was the silent conductor of the orchestra, bringing a new melody to my life. Religion teaches us that we are in control of the process. But we are not. We dream, plan, and measure each step. But He is in you, disclosing hidden riches in the darkness. He will give you access to His vault filled with wisdom so you can complete every mission. Go mining for that hidden cache inside you as if you were searching for silver and gold. It's hidden for you, not from you. It will take courage and faith. Rise when you don't feel like rising. Stand up when you don't feel like standing. Get back in the ring and fight for life. Fortune favors the brave.

On November 6, 2016, I wrote: I'm so happy to be at the deer lease again in nature, with God, family, friends. It's wonderful to spend time with Addison and Tim. This is opening weekend of white-tail deer season.

I had worked persistently to build up my upper-body strength following a bilateral mastectomy. I wanted to get back to the deer lease and hunt. My goal was to be able to lift and accurately aim my heavy rifle. I designed and implemented a course of action. Regularly participating in Tai Chi classes, gently working out with light weights, and walking, I focused on increasing my overall strength, stamina, and mobility following surgery and amid chemotherapy treatments. It was vital for me to set goals. My hard work paid off. Opening weekend of whitetail deer season was three months following surgery and a few days following my third chemotherapy treatment. Don and I were together that day in the deer stand. I watched through the binoculars as the deer came into view. Raising my rifle, I gently pulled the trigger, landing a nice eight-point buck and lots of meat to carry us through the winter. We have so many memories hunting together. I was so happy and so proud that I had achieved my goal in the middle of the crisis. Establish challenging, purposeful objectives. Set a course of action. Keep moving forward with intentionality until you successfully cross the finish line.

The next morning I wrote: Being at the lease allows me lots of quiet time. I am in Hebrews, deeply meditating on each chapter. Jesus speaks to us through His recorded words and actions. His blood still speaks. He is my Apostle and My High Priest. I hear His voice as He speaks today. The author of Hebrews admonishes,

Today if you will hear His voice.
From Hebrews 3:15 NKJV.

I choose to listen and hear. He is still speaking better things, a new covenant, a new relationship. He suffered everything we endure in this life so that He can have compassion for our pain and sorrow. When we hurt, we are sharing in His deeply grievous trials. We can identify with Him. We know He has already experienced it for us and is going through it with us. He took it all on Himself in His life and His death. He took all that agony on Himself for us. He can identify with us, understand us, have compassion on us, and save us. He gives us grace to stand and withstand all. He is our faithful High Priest that has passed from death to life. He took it all to His Father in His life, His death, and His resurrection. What He took to the Father was compressed into liquid love, grace, and more mercy than you can imagine. You can stand tall and bear all as you advance into that place of grace. He is well-able to sustain you. He will keep you from falling and lift you. Look up. Your deliverance is drawing near. Look into His face of compassion, love, and power. Only a faithful high priest who has passed from death to life can do that. He has even conquered death, so it does not have a sting and does not win.

But emotions swing wide and carry me for a ride. Suddenly that hairy scary specter appears again. I look around our fifth-wheel at the deer lease. I see so many signs that I used to have hair. I thought I had already processed this. Hair clips, headbands, bobby pins, hairbrushes, combs, etc. are in every drawer and cabinet. These reminders make me sad and sick inside. I want this to all be over. I want my hair and health back. I want my breast back, reconstructive surgery done. These expanders are uncomfortable, and I don't like to look at my breastless self.

I blinked my eyes and snapped back to stability. I had purchased a new camouflage-patterned scarf to wear at the lease to royally adorn my hairless head. I wrapped it securely and crowned myself like a princess, while sporting my camo insulated overalls. I had wound the scarf around my head like a Swamy's turban. As we were leaving to hunt that afternoon, Addison said, "Mimi, I like your camouflage scarf." My heart melted. My grandson knows how to make my heart sing a happy song! Sometimes the simplest, sweet words are amplified in a crisis.

Getting around the deer lease was not easy. The effects of the chemotherapy treatments were cumulative, meaning they each added up and intensified accordingly. I had just had my third. My heart was weak, and I was tired all the time. The least exertion left me out of breath. Each time we went hunting, Addison took all of us to our deer stand in the golf cart. When I say 'in,' I mean in, on, around - anywhere we could load a hunter and our rifles. There were about seven of us loaded on the small cart. Usually, Addison would drop each of us off within eye-shot of our deer stand. We would have to walk the rest of the way. I did not have the energy to walk very far while carrying my heavy rifle. One day we were having trouble with the battery on the cart. We were concerned it did not have the power to go the entire distance, taking each person close to their stands. I expressed my concern at the prospect of them having to walk so far to their stand if the cart battery gave out. Addison said, "The most important thing is to get you and Papa to your stand." He knew I had little stamina. I love Addison and his caring heart.

Chapter 23

CHEMO CHANGE

On November 7, 2016 Don and I met with Dr. Usrey. We had been meeting with him every two weeks. My schedule with oncology was that I would receive chemotherapy one week then meet with him the next. Before each chemotherapy infusion, the lab would draw lots and lots of blood, test it to see if I was healthy enough for the chemo delivery, then, once approved, I would lay back in a recliner for two to three hours as that sweet cancer killer was delivered to my body through the PICC line in my left arm. Now it was time to switch to a different chemotherapy formula that included Taxol. The side effects would be different from 'the red devil'- not as harsh as the Adriamycin I had been receiving. However, there could be an infusion reaction that included hot flashes, skin redness, rash, trouble breathing. It could increase my neuropathy, which had already caused numbness in my fingertips, ankles, and feet. The neuropathy persists today, sometimes affecting balance and my ability to hold on to things. Sometimes it's hardly noticeable. The effects wax and wane. With Taxol, I would experience less fatigue and nausea than with the previous chemotherapy formula.

Taxol (Paclitaxel) chemo days were different. First, I was given a Benadryl drip to diminish the Taxol side effects. The Benadryl made me loose as a goose - actually kind of a fun, peaceful, tipsy feeling. My words were slurred and my gait was unsteady. I needed help getting to the bathroom during chemo treatment. Some patients slept during the Benadryl delivery, but I did not want to miss any part of my life. I had learned to embrace and savor every moment. I drifted a bit occasionally, but I did not sleep. By the time chemotherapy was over, I was at myself again. After about three hours of infusion, I was back home working in my home office.

Fun with friends kept me going. During nearly four months of chemotherapy, I did not get out much except for physician visits. My energy was low, and my immune system was compromised. I did not mingle among crowds, risking exposure to sickness. When friends or family came to visit, Don and I were always delighted, and it lifted our spirits. On November 8, 2016, our good friends Mike and Martha Wedemeyer came to visit. We watched the presidential election results together. We chattered on and on as we devoured Don's delicious, barbecued ribs. I appreciated sharing my situation, my story, my song with Martha. A shared burden is a lighter load. Dear Reader, people need to know about your journey so they can help you and others. Friends always promise to be there for each other through it all.

My relentless pursuit of purpose pushed me forward. Knowing the meaning of my being had always fueled my internal fire. The meditations of my heart November 2016:

Sometimes, I see my dreams wasting away. I'm suspended, disconnected from life's flow. I see a puzzle with the mosaic of my purpose forged on it. I am one piece of the puzzle, but I'm detached from the whole. All the scattered puzzle pieces are there and will be moved into place. Father, I see Your hand joining the pieces in Your time, for Your purpose. You are choosing each puzzle piece with intention, monitoring each move. The puzzle pieces will snap into place. I will be whole again. I'll write the vision when I see it and run with courage, joy, and sweet abandon.

I welcomed support from people who had been through cancer diagnosis before me. On November 9, 2016, I spoke with Tim's friend, Lisa Jones. I thanked her for the gifts she sent. She had been through breast cancer treatment and was so encouraging. She told me about her experience with radiation and some personal tips - do the exercises they give you and rub your armpits with fresh aloe vera juice. She advised that the aloe vera juice would prevent scarring and discoloration. She also recommended acupuncture for inflammation and pain. Her doctor at MD Anderson Cancer Center had recommended it.

Work was a great distraction from my present circumstances. I was grateful to have a job where I could work at home. I was also thankful for times of peace and rest. On November 13, 2016, we returned to the deer lease. All I could do was rest. The cumulative treatment side effects had taken their toll. I rested in our fifth-wheel, reading, meditating on God's word and enjoying nature.

Let me hear of Your unfailing love each morning, for I am trusting in You.
From Psalm 143:8 NLT

Chapter 24

PERPLEXING RADIATION CONSULTATION

On November 16, 2016, Don and I consulted with the radiology oncologist. Dr. Usrey, our oncologist, had recommended radiation therapy following my eight rounds of chemotherapy. I was not too sure I wanted to go through with that. I studied information from alternative, complementary, and natural methods of healing and prevention of recurrence and trusting God. Just to be transparent here, I was not in the mood to visit another doctor who would probably recommend the traditional physician pathway based on statistical data. I did not want to do anything else to my body that might cause collateral damage. Some medical cancer treatments can also cause unintended harm to other parts of the body and body systems. Collateral damage is any death, injury, or further damage that is an unintended result of military operations. You may hit the intended target, but other things may also get damaged. I was also studying medical statistical data and realized that the physicians were making recommendations based on statistical outcome studies alone, and they could not give me any guarantees. Today our consultation with this particular radiation oncologist was very disappointing and disturbing. He was entirely objective and emotionally disengaged.

I was not impressed with our conversation. I thought, 'This is my body and my life we are talking about.' Of course, he was recommending radiation therapy. When I pressed him with questions, he answered each one but was somewhat irritated with my query. He reluctantly gave each answer. He explained that radiation therapy was a insurance policy. He warned that if I did not have radiation therapy, there was a 25% chance cancer would reoccur. If I opted to have the recommended radiation therapy, there was a 12% chance of cancer returning. He wanted to radiate the chest wall where cancer had been on the right side and where the cancer had been cut out. He also wanted to deliver radiation to the under arm on the same side where the four sentinel nodes had been removed. His plan was to give thirty days, five days a week, radiation therapy with no breaks except for the weekend. He explained that side effects would include red, irritated skin like sunburn and that I would be tired. What was so new about being tired? I thought. He continued to report that there is a sliver of the lung that's hit by the radiation, but he did not believe that it was a big deal. They were not his lungs. When I pressed him with more questions, he finally relented with a surprising response. "We over-treat a lot of people, and we don't know who they are." Finally, the bottom-line truth. That answer was alarming to me. I did not want to be one of those over-treated people, but how could I be sure? It has been reported that a high percentage of oncologists would not take the course of treatment they recommend and deliver to their patients. In the cancer world, physicians are bound by standards of care that they must follow. There are variations or choices within that pathway, but they are bound to follow the path set by standard practice guidelines. So they recommend, then you decide. Basically, the statement rolling around in your head is 'do or die?' Does a Monopoly board include 'Uneasy Street?' If so, I'm on it.

Fighting the good fight, I quietly combatted every voice that might cause me to fall apart. I punched and counterpunched to maintain a strong and stable mind. I would win each skirmish on my terms. My dwelling place was the love of God.

Keep yourselves in the love of God, looking for the mercy of our Lord Jesus Christ unto eternal life.
From Jude 1:21 NKJV.

The word of God is alive and powerful. 'Keep yourselves in the love of God' meant so much to me. Holy Spirit brought that to my heart with joy, peace, power, and instruction like I had not felt in a while. Keeping, preserving, staying power for each hour. I wrote:

I feel so kept. I love my God and I love people and God loves me and God loves the world and all the people in it. Choose life. That God-kind of life has a positive charge and has a more abundant, creative force than you can ever imagine. My armament will be the love of God. I will adamantly advance toward victory. Father God, You make me brave.

Faithful, friendly phone calls lifted my spirits. On November 23, 2016, my friend Karen and I had a great phone visit. She relayed that she had a dream the week of November 21. In the dream, she was talking to God and me. She told me, "Give me some of that (referring to my cancer) so I can share it with you and receive what God is giving you and get some of it off of you." I know it sounds strange, but she reported it as a good thing. She believed God was working great things in me - spirit, soul, and body. She believed I would share it with the world one day. She received 'it,' and declared it as a privilege. She said, "Lord, don't leave me behind." She said, "Jeanie, what if God is calling us to war, and we must have each other's back." She talked about being sure-footed. As the dream continued, God told us not to lose our 'sparkle'. In Genesis 2:10 the Hebrew name for river is 'nahor'. It comes from a primitive word that means 'sparkle' or 'to be cheerful'. In the Bible, rivers are frequently metaphors of the life-giving presence of God. I shared that what she was doing in the dream, taking on my cancer, was what Jesus did on the cross. He took our sin, sickness, sorrow, disappointments, and grief. He took it upon Himself when He was on the cross. I told Karen she was sharing in His divine nature. I was not fighting this fight alone. A great cloud of witnesses surrounded me, and Karen was one of them.

Run your race. Don't compare yourself with others. I was more determined than ever to keep myself in the love of God. God challenged Job out of the whirlwind, "Do you know the laws of heaven?" True wisdom knows when to speak and when to be silent. I knew my story was not over. The last word was yet to be uttered. There was a lot more going on in my darkness than I could imagine. God was opening me up to diverse, unique perspectives. On November 28, 2016, I wrote:

God created me to be a life-giving, pro-creative force in this universe. I will live as You created me to be. The creative, generative power of God lives in me. I am a partaker of His divine nature.

Now more medical intervention was being suggested. On December 5, 2016, at our bi-weekly visit with Dr. Usrey, he proposed a hormone-blocking medication following radiation therapy. I could not believe there was more to this cancer medical intervention. The good news just kept unfolding - NOT! He said the type of cancer I had was 94% estrogen receptor-positive. That means my cancer cells thrived on the hormone, estrogen. Taking the estrogen hormone-blocking medication would starve any remaining cancer cells. I explained that my ovaries had been removed years ago. I probably had no estrogen in my body. He explained that fat cells and adrenal glands also produce estrogen. I was now learning about cancer stem cells.

MedlinePlus.gov, a part of the National Institute of Health U.S. National Library of Medicine, defines stem cells as cells with the ability to develop into many other types of cells in the body. According to the National Institute of Health National Library of Medicine at PubMed.gov, breast cancer is still the most common malignancy in women. One of the reasons patients succumb to breast cancer is treatment resistance leading to metastasis and recurrence. A cancer stem cell is a cell within a tumor that is capable of self-renewal. I learned that breast cancer stem cells could still be hiding in my body even after surgically carving it out of my breast, chemo chemical warfare, and Darth Vader Lightsaber targeted radiation. There is no way to detect breast cancer stem cells. Oh my, so much to research. I was also learning to let food be my medicine, a part of my treatment protocol. There were natural, God-given ways to discourage cancer stem cells' growth and to support healthy cell development.

Chapter 25

FROM SUFFERING TO SHARPER VISION

You will never possess what you are unwilling to pursue. I was now experiencing God's re-visioning. I was getting a divine make-over. My assignment was unfolding daily. As people came to my mind, I would pray for them. My mission continued to be teaching and preaching, but with a different expression - writing. I was to promoted wellness by producing and selling my Well Within products. The wisdom and words that were emerging amazed me. He told me, 'Keep your eyes and ears open as the road less traveled emerges in front of you. It will rise and become the high road.' On December 21, 2016, the Holy Spirit said, 'I want to commune with you.' I was in my bed reading a book. I turned out the lights and shut down everything. Jesus came to my bed-side. I could not see His face. He was clothed in a linen robe with a hood, like a shepherd's cloak. We communicated with unspoken love, comfort, and closeness. He clothed me with His robe. I found myself standing beside Him. He clasped my hand, and we began to walk forward. I knew that He was walking with me into my future. His rod and His staff continued to comfort me.

The final chemical weapon was being deployed. December 21, 2016 was my last chemotherapy treatment. Yes, I know what you are thinking. Right before Christmas. Can't we catch a break here? No. But I was ready to have this part of my life behind me. We had celebrated Christmas with Tim and his family the previous weekend. We then traveled to Tomball to spend Christmas Eve and Day with my son Brian, River, and Catherine. We all went out to eat at our favorite Asian restaurant on Christmas Eve and had a great time. Then Don and I returned to our hotel room and spent a meaningful Christmas Eve together, just the two of us. That night we thanked God over and over for what He had brought us through. With great joy, we had a quiet celebration of life, talking, and watching old movies. I will never forget that special celebration we had together. We were so happy. The next day, Christmas Day, we spent at Brian's house. We had a great dinner and visited with Catherine's mother, sister, and family. Brian is a gourmet chef, and Catherine is the best sous-chef de cuisine. Even though I was not feeling my best, being with family and friends brought great contentment and joy and nullified any negative feelings in my body. I can't explain the new gladness and love I was experiencing, knowing God had led us this far and would continue to usher us into the future.

That evening we drove to my sister Alene's house in Burton and enjoyed a grand celebration of life. Our cousin, John, and his wife, Candy, from Mobile, came to visit. I will never forget the love and compassion in John's eyes as he looked at me, with my bald head wrapped in a sassy, colorful scarf. Such love and caring came straight to my heart from my cousin that day. Love is a powerful thing!

Then we traveled on to the deer lease, a place of fun, rest, peace, and time in nature. Tim and his family stayed with us. Unwrapping my scarf in private, I showed Melissa my bald head. I did not do that with many people. My hair had been such an intimate part of me all my life. I had loved my hair. At that time, I did not even like to look at myself in the mirror.

As promised, in early January, my hair started growing back. I was being crowned with new glory. Each day following my last chemotherapy treatment, I would look for signs of new growth. Finally, fine fuzz began to emerge. It was a small sign of victory, but it was a promise of more to come. Then one Saturday morning, when Don was away for the weekend, I saw a bit of hair. When I say a bit, I mean a nubbin! I almost needed a magnifying glass to see it. I was so excited but was not sure what to think about it. It was white. I had colored my hair since I was 16 years old and did not know my natural color. Suddenly, my daughter-in-law, Melissa, came through the front door. I told her my hair had started growing back and asked if she wanted to see it. We went to the bathroom with a large mirror and lots of light. I removed the scarf and unveiled my scalp with at teeny tiny bit of hair. You could barely see it. She got excited and exclaimed, "It's beautiful." She was one of my biggest cheerleaders. I touched it and frowned. Looking back in the mirror, I moaned, "But Melissa, it's white!" She responded, "But Jean, what if it's blonde?" We laughed. That was the first realization that my hair might be coming in white, gray, or both.

As my strands sprouted, ever so slowly, I gradually stopped covering it. My silver locks in front gradually gave way to gray in the back. A friend told me that young people were bleaching their hair and coloring it gray and silver. Isn't it just like God to give me chic, radiant tresses? One day our family was sitting on the patio. I looked at my son, Tim, and noticed his hair's naturally white and gray pattern. I exclaimed, "Tim, my hair looks just like yours!" He responded, "But Mom, what if my hair looks just like yours?" I was so proud of that moment, having my son note that our hair color blueprint was the same - personally designed by God.

Chapter 26

MYSTERY TO MASTERY

If it had not been the Lord who was on our side...
From Psalm 124 :1 KJV.

But what about those who continue to suffer with seemingly no rescue? I have always been troubled when people proclaimed that God had answered prayers when things were going right. But words like 'blessed, blessing, answered prayer' are never used to describe people enduring hardship, sorrow, pain, and death. God is always on our side in sickness and health through the valley and on the mountaintop. He is with us at conception, birth, and death. In our transition to the heavenly realm (death) or our sustained stay on the earth, He is always for us and never against us.

He has the keys to death.
From Revelations 1:18 NAS.

If I am to transition from the earth through the shadow of death to the heavenly realm, it will be on His terms in His timing and not anyone else's. I grew to trust Him more every day with all of my life - all seasons, life events, relationships, timing, sickness, and death.

On January 22, 2017, I wrote:

You cannot do hand-to-hand combat with fear with your own human devices. When initially diagnosed, God led me to face fear first. I purposefully got in the ring and faced my opponent. I let trust rise and prevail. The word of God is growing in me. Get quiet and be still. Know that He alone is God. He has not toppled off the throne just because you are going through a threatening storm. He will speak in your stillness and your smallness. Trust in His profound word. His alive word will carry you through to the next round in the ring. Prepare to block the next blow.

I refuse to watch from the sidelines as others play life. By February 10, 2017, I was learning to run my own race. Sometimes we live life with a quiet vigilance, considering how we might fit into other people's agendas and expectations. We look in their eyes like a mirror for feedback. When their expression whispers disapproval, we flinch back and morph, yielding to their design. I was learning to be me in the midst of a people that long for approval. Some people withhold their blessing when we don't obey their quiet demands to conform. We perform to earn their social permission to take the next step. We quickly calculate in our minds what they want to see, then do it. I decided to live life unedited, free to be me with lots of adventure, joy, and life.

Sometimes the best decisions come out of the worst circumstances. Limitations were lifting, but the minefield of my mind was exploding. It was populated with treasure-filled aspirations guarded by threatening thought-bombs. I began to feel a nudge to write, but several concerns jumbled my thoughts. I had multiple fanciful dreams. They came to me like previews on a movie screen. I began to write and prioritize them. I knew if I obeyed that inner voice, the ideas would never stop. If I did not start, the creativity would dry up and never flow again. I would be forever disappointed in myself for not stepping out. My second concern was the lack of discretionary time. I worked more than 40 hours a week and had a full-time husband. I was and will ever be devoted to him. I called my cousin, Sylvia, who is a seasoned author, speaker, and publisher. I told her about my need to write and briefed her on some of my ideas. She confirmed that people needed to hear what I had to say. She, too, has a full-time husband whom she loves deeply. She said most of the time she wrote before he got up in the morning. There were also times when she said, "I've got to go write." She encouraged me to draw a line on the calendar - the beginning. Then say 'no' to everything that does not support your writing project. She advised that I obey when God says, "I have a message that I want the community-at-large to hear." I later learned that everybody has a story, and there is always someone out there who needs to hear it. Another contrary missile I had to overcome was, "Who do you think you are?" Who was I to say I had something to offer by putting my name on a book's cover? What made me think I could become an author? Another thought-bomb was that I knew nothing about writing or publishing. I had enjoyed my work as a speech-language pathologist and had learned a lot about the healthcare industry, but authoring a book was a whole new arena. What if I fail? But, Dear Reader, what if you fly?

Let the new you ascend. Dare to be what you've never been before. On February 12, 2017, I began to overcome each thought-bomb and started writing for an audience of one, myself. My fingers danced across the keyboard of my computer. Day by day, I wrote in the snatches of time I could steal. The words came fast and steady. The flow felt good. I began to research authoring and publishing online. I first created a devotional for our church camp counseling group. The camp board of directors asked me to create a series of devotionals to inspire our camp counselors. The devotional helped each counselor meditate on God's word and spend time with Him. Each day's devotional included an assignment to help the counselor support each camper they would encounter.

I later found a publisher, Eddie Smith, owner and CEO of Worldwide Publishing Group. He encouraged and coached me as I finished an entire book. He mentored me from words on a page to a book available on Amazon and other sites. He coaxed me to expand my ideas, helped me find and correct my mistakes. He helped with cover design ideas. I could not have done it without his guidance. My first book, *Mindful Meditation: 30 Days Uniting With The Heart of God*, is now published, and I am currently writing my second book. Many of my friends have said, "I did not know you had it in you." The truth is, I didn't either. I just put one foot out in from of the other, following the inner voice. I ignored small, intimidating thoughts and moved forward each day. I believed I could do it, no matter what. I still have more ideas that I want to pursue. Dear Reader, do you have a dream? Does it seem out of reach right now? Does it seem far away? You can do it. Listen to that inner voice, trust God, and follow the path He sets before you. It is not always easy. Don't be afraid to choose the hard way. Life always emerges out of the darkness. Let innovation, energy, and new design surface like a mighty submarine out of your troubled waters. Your valley is not your finale. If you shoot for the moon and miss, even then you'll be among the stars.

Chapter 27

ROCKING, REELING, AND WORKING IT OUT

I'm now entering the radiation zone. Strange how you just keep following the path the cancer industry maps out for you. I had consulted with my husband and my sons, Brian and Tim, at every juncture. I needed their counsel. I was learning many natural pathways to healing, but I dared not make a decision regarding my health that did not have their input. I needed their support along the way and heeded their advice. Even though I did my research, spoke with others who had walked this road, looked at the data that included how much longer you might live if you choose this pathway or that, the journey was full of hard choices.

Near the end of my recent chemotherapy treatment, I had gone for my first consultation with the radiation oncologist to discuss radiation therapy. Remember? That visit was a disaster. Now it's the end of February 2017, and tomorrow, March 1, 2017, I will start radiation therapy. Last week I had gone for my second consultation with a new radiation oncologist and was 'marked for life' with tattoos to define the perimeters of radiation-targeted beams. The tattoos were permanent, small dots designed to guide the radiation machine. I asked the radiology tech if she would create and place some tatted nipples on my bare chest. (Sorry. That was an overshare!) She laughed and said she was not that good at tatting. Things proceeded, and I got marked with the 'dot' tattoos and some 'sharpie' marks. A few days later, I got a call from radiology saying they were ready to get started. Following a brief reprieve, things were becoming real again. Fear crouched near as I considered the possible side effects, both immediate and future. Tears came to my eyes. Yet I looked at how far God had brought us. I say 'us' because Don and I, together, had faced the horrors and debilitation of mastectomy and chemotherapy. We had fought like champions. We did everything we could to stand, withstand, and overcome. Now we were more united than ever. We were fearless. And now, we were facing another giant - radiation therapy. While worry wanted to wear us down, we were ascending on angels' wings.

Radiation is defined as the process in which beams of intense energy are used to kill cancer cells. As I pondered radiation's definition, I began to think about creation and how God created science laws. He created light. Visible light must travel through the invisible structures and physics elements that God designed and built to work according to His blueprint. I wrote:

> Tonight I will meditate on the laws of God that we call science. I will especially meditate on light and its power in the hands of God! Tomorrow, as I enter the radiation arena and lay down for treatment, I will see God as He emits and plans the route of the power that comes from the machines created by man, but powered by God.

I knew it was come-back time. I allowed myself to do what I had done before. I let God turn my setback into a win instead of a wait.

A righteous man may fall seven times and rise again.
From Proverbs 24:16 NKJ.

When your situation is breaking down, God is breaking through. Breakup erupts into a breakout. See your obstacle as an opportunity. It's time for you to push and sustain your best mental and emotional effort. You must be willing to pay the price. Focus on God and His calling alone. Maintain that center, pleasing Him and Him alone.

Big girls and boys do cry. Dear Reader, I must bear my heart here. I want you to understand that it's okay to cry. I experienced depths of emotions throughout my experience that I had not known before. I felt filleted like a fish with its guts hanging out. I was overflowing with new heights of joy and laugher as never before. God was hollowing me out and filling me with a full spectrum of genuine, authentic feelings. My emotions were no longer bridled. The cork had popped off the champagne bottle, and all life was spewing forth with pure, sweet abandon. It felt good to be fully me.

But the first day of radiation, as brave as I was and full of positive affirmations, tears started rolling down my cheeks as they laid me on that cold, steel table. I hated the thought of damaging my body with radiation. My bare, breastless chest faced upward for all the world to see. They pulled the radiation-emitting equipment over me and into a precise position. The radiology technician left the room. He watched through a small window, setting the computer to work its magic according to the prescribed route and duration. Tears flowed the entire time as the monstrous machinery moved within its computer-guided boundaries, painlessly blasting my right upper-chest and armpit - about seven long minutes. I got up from the table and apologized for the tears. The technicians were quite supportive. That was the last time I cried during radiation treatment. From then on, I walked in, bared my chest, and laid down like a fearless, powerful princess. In the waiting room each day, I brought joy, love, and support to each person sweating it out with me.

Wonder Woman, the Warrior Princess, was emerging. In April 2017, weeks after I had completed radiation, I went to a Spiderman movie with my grandson, Andrew. Peter Parker was learning to embrace his newly discovered powers and adopt his new identity as Spiderman, champion of the people. He was challenged as he anticipated engaging impossible situations with his recently discovered superpowers. On the outside, he was Peter Parker. As a young boy, he had been orphaned when his parents were killed in a plane crash. An aunt and uncle raised him. As a teenager, his secret superpowers started to emerge. He began to learn to use his mysterious, hidden powers to fight evil. On the inside, he was Spiderman. He was indeed a new creature - a dual being. He learned to fight and overcome the forces of darkness, not only for himself but also for others. As Peter Parker, he was often scared. But when a higher purpose grabbed hold of him, he became a superhero. On the way home from the movie, I told Andrew that we are becoming superheroes with superpowers. He said, "Mimi, how can we do that?" I told him, "We are God's new creations with His superpowers to overcome evil!"

The best of times and the worst of times come to us all. Be ready to endure harsh seasons. Tough times are temporary and only last until the opening of the next episode. If you think you can't, you can, through Christ who gives you incredible grit and determination to undergo, overcome, and walk out better on the other side. Part of the perseverance process is learning to cry out to God. Praise Him when you don't feel like it, hope when you are tempted to give up, believe when you are afraid of being disappointed, and be brutally honest with God and yourself. The apostle Paul endured and focused on the mission in the face of much physical pain, fear of death, disappointment with people, and rejection by those God sent him to rescue. A dear soldier is a warrior on the front lines of battle facing fear and death. His commanding officer loves him and knows his potential from the inside out. Some of you have known physical pain and mental anguish you thought you could not endure, but you did. You've been discouraged by the circumstances of your life. You are disappointed with yourself and with God. He tenderly sees you as His dearly beloved soldier. He has not forgotten you or cast you aside. Your purpose still resides and will ever abide in you. Turn your devastation into an adventure. Advance in the face of push-back. Dare to dream the impossible dream. Reach higher than you've ever reached before.

Chapter 28

CAREGIVER PERSPECTIVE

Interview with My Husband, Don

Me: What thoughts and emotions did you experience when you first heard me say, 'I just got back from a follow-up mammogram, and they think it's cancer.'

Don: Just shock. My first emotions were just shock. I knew to pray - that it did not have to be true just because they 'thought it was.' We tried to comfort each other the best we could and get our thoughts together. It was a devastating message that it could be cancer. It was a total, knock-down shock. Jeanie had always been healthy. We had never faced anything like this. You start wondering and praying. What are we going to do? What's our next step? I was in total shock. It broke my heart. I cried. We cried. It was a bad situation, a real bad situation. We were facing the worst problem in our 46 years of marriage, except the loss of loved ones through the years. Jeanie and I discussed what route we wanted to take - Tyler physicians or MD Anderson Cancer Center in Houston. A few days later, I went to get a pedicure. While Taylor was giving me a pedicure, I told him the situation we were going through. Someone had told us about Dr. Fender. A lady sitting in the chair next to me got up to pay, turned, and said, "You don't have to go anywhere. You can stay right here. I had breast cancer, and Dr. Fender was my doctor. We ended up getting some of the best doctors.

The rest of the time, I took care of my wife. I cooked, cleaned, and drove her everywhere she needed to go. We went through some tough times. Jeanie went through thinking about alternate routes of treatment. I felt the best decision would be to take the physicians' advice and the steps they recommended. I knew God was working in her body and her life. Every time the oncologist would look at her blood work, he would marvel.

Some moments I would get emotional and pray and cry, mostly at night when I went to bed. I would get emotional but not in front of her.

Don: You must hear the hair story. I would see her combing her hair in the back yard, and hair was flying everywhere. Finally, I told her, "Let me just shave it off." She agreed, and I put her in a chair in the backyard and cut it close then shaved it off. She laughed and cried, and we talked throughout that entire event. Then she started wearing scarves wrapped around her head. She looked like a fortune-teller. She kept telling everyone to get her a crystal ball, tarot cards, and a palm-reading instruction book for Christmas. Everyone seemed to love the scarves.

Me: What about the mastectomy?

Don: It came time for the surgery. We had decided she was going to have both breasts removed. A lot of our friends came to the hospital the morning of surgery. Each doctor came and prayed with Jeanie before surgery. The anesthesiologist also prayed with us. God was with us. He was with everyone involved. God had a plan.

During surgery, the doctors kept us posted. The plastic surgeon finally came out and said he had put the expanders in. She stayed in recovery for quite a long time. We finally got her settled into the room. I was so concerned. Recovery in the hospital was rough, and that kept me torn up. After a few days, she came home, and I took good care of her. All of our church friends visited and brought us food for over two weeks. Our friend, Lou Ann, organized all that. We could not have made it without the support of our friends. Jeanie's sister, Alene, a nurse, came and stayed with us for a week. She took care of Jeanie's bandages, drain tubes, etc.. She helped with things that would have been very difficult for me to do. We could not have made it without her help.

I would hate to think of anyone going through a situation like this without God in their life. We went through every step with Him seeing us through.

Me: Talk about our doctors.

Don: Dr. Harrison was one of our best supporters - emotionally and spiritually. He is the most wonderful plastic surgeon that ever lived. He kept us encouraged with things that he did and things that he said. Talking through the diagnosis, he reminded us, 'Your house is not on fire.'

He educated us about mastectomy and breast reconstruction and started throwing silicone implants at me, saying, "There! How does that feel?"

He came to check Jeanie the morning after surgery and found a heart monitor on her. He was upset. "What is this? Who put this on you? Why did they put it on you? I am so angry." Jeanie explained that her blood pressure had gone down during the night, and they wanted to monitor her heart. He sent for the nurse and asked why she did it. She told him. He told her he was always available throughout the night and to call him anytime they needed him. We always felt confident that Dr. Harrison would take care of us. He wanted everything to be perfect for his patients.

Me: What advice would you give to the person wanting to help someone get through a situation like this?

Don: 1. Trust your heart and soul to God. 2. Don't let your wife know what you are going through emotionally. 3. Do all you can to encourage her. Tell her that she is going to be okay and that you will be with her throughout. Keep her spirits up. 4. Do everything you can to take care of her - big and small. 5. Make sure she has everything she needs. 6. During the chemotherapy treatments, her thinking may get slow and her memory poor. Just stay positive when it happens. Let her know that doctors said this would be part of it, and everything will be fine. 7. Let her know you are there for her day and night.

A Conversation with My Sister, Alene

Me: Alene, what thoughts went through your head when I called you with the news that the doctor thought I had breast cancer?

Alene: I never thought about Jeanie dying before. A few years back, I had been diagnosed with thyroid cancer and had my thyroid removed. With my kind of cancer, you just fix it and move on with life. I thought about our cousin, Jeannie, who had died of breast cancer many years ago. You expect people in your life to be there forever. Just like landscape changes, nothing in your life stays the same. People-landscape changes also. Then you start thinking about yourself. Every bump and lump makes you start imagining you have something wrong with your body.

I watched Jeanie persist from diagnosis, through all debilitating treatments and fears. She was able to redirect her thoughts and tell her body, 'you can do this.' There is something exceptional about the one who can persevere.

Chapter 29

QUESTION, QUEST, CONQUEST

There is an unsettled question that has persisted throughout eternity. Does God cause calamity or death? Does God bring heartache or confusion? Ask Job. Some scholars believe that the Book of Job was written before any other book of the Bible. Job's dark season was long, grievous, and unyielding. Job asked many questions and expressed his profound agony of body and soul. But he endured hard times. In the face of deep heartache, physical pain, and profound grief, Job said,

> *But as for me, I know that my Redeemer lives, and that He will stand on the earth at last. And I know that after this body has decayed, this body shall see God. Then He will be on my side! Yes, I shall see him, not as a stranger, but as a friend! What a glorious hope!*
> From Job 19:25-27 TLB.

The closer you get to death, the more you yearn to see Him. Your priorities begin to shift. Each moment of life becomes precious. Before time began, before the great disruption, God created a place of peace. Then chaos came. God arose, and step-by-step began making order out of devastation, one day at a time. God did not get in a hurry. He is in charge of your process. He is building something great in you that you could not have erected on your own. The order you had created in your life was blown apart. Now God has become the architect, custom builder, and construction foreman. He is molding you from the inside out. You are becoming a champion of His grace. By faith, Abraham went where God led, even when he did not know where he was going. He was looking forward to a city with foundations whose maker and builder is God. By faith, Moses left the riches and comforts of Egypt and followed the plan of God. It was not easy to leave the life of a prince he had forsaken in Egypt. He learned how to endure hard times by going through them. Each hardship unveiled wisdom and resources he did not know he had. Don't witlessly weaken and wander through who, what, when, where, why? Assess the situation and respond with unrelenting determination. Ask how and what next.

Map your own highway to healing and health. When first diagnosed, I explored all options, both conventional and nonconventional. I asked my healthcare professionals many questions and took notes in my journal at each visit. I learned that not all breast cancers are the same. I researched the possible causes of cancer. I found that many oncology professionals do not concern themselves with causative or contributing factors. Most of their focus is on treatment options based on each unique diagnosis, risks associated with those options, and statistical outcomes based on their treatment. What is cancer? Cancer is a complex group of diseases with many causes. It is the disease that results when cellular changes cause the uncontrolled growth and division of cells. But what causes cellular changes or injury? Hypoxia (decreased oxygen), ischemia (reduced blood flow), physical and chemical agents, radiation and toxins, metabolic abnormalities (genetic or acquired), immune dysfunction (hypersensitivity reactions and autoimmune disease), aging, and nutritional imbalances. Cell damage or injury can be caused by various changes or stress that a cell suffers due to external or internal environmental changes. Substances that cause cancer are called carcinogens. Causes may include environmental agents, viral, or genetic factors. Changes may be due to exposure to cancer-causing substances. In most cases, cancer can't be attributed to a single cause.

After a focused inquiry into possible contributing factors to my cancer, I decided to change a few things at a time. As I mentioned before, I needed to reduce my toxic load. Toxic load refers to the accumulation of toxins and chemicals in our bodies that we ingest, absorb through our skin, or breathe. It includes the food we eat, the water we drink, and the personal care and household products we use. I looked closely at the skincare products I was using. I had always bought the most expensive products and used them diligently. I had often laughingly told my husband that I would never retire because I always wanted to be able to buy expensive, anti-aging skincare products. Boy, was I ever wrong here. I found out that the skincare line I was using included carcinogens. I immediately stopped using them and threw them away - a lot of money dumped in the trash. I considered several natural commercial skincare lines. My search also led me to develop my personally-designed skincare recipes. I got a bright idea to do a little market research on myself and family members. As we tried each product, I refined the formula to improve outcomes. I gradually perfected my recipes and now market them as Well Within skincare products. I developed a face scrub that people love. I make it fresh and sell locally at a low cost. Well Within also includes body powder and other items. I make my own toothpaste and deodorant. Everything I put on my body is natural and contains essential oils that nurture and support good health.

The next thing I researched was our public drinking water. My review of the chemicals in our drinking water was quite revealing. Typical tap water contains chlorine, fluoride compounds, and trihalomethanes (TMHs). You are also likely to find salts of arsenic, radium, aluminum, copper, lead, mercury, and cadmium. Hormones, nitrates, and pesticides are probably flowing through your faucet. My findings were alarming. At first, I started drinking bottled water, filtered by reverse osmosis, and stored in BPA-free plastic containers. BPA, bisphenol A, is an industrial chemical that has been used since the 1960s to make certain plastics and resins. BPA has xenoestrogen-mimicking, hormone-like properties. Now I only use bottled water for traveling. I purchased a countertop Berkey water purification system for my home drinking and cooking water.

Because most of our fruits and vegetables are grown in nutrient-depleted soil and sprayed with pesticides, I decided to purchase only organically-grown fruits and vegetables when possible. The meat industry raises animals in feedlots and chicken houses. They feed small doses of antibiotics to animals daily, causing them to gain 3% more weight than without antibiotics. Remember, profits in the meat industry are measured by weight. According to the World Health Organization (WHO), overuse and misuse of antibiotics in animals and humans contribute to antibiotic resistance's rising threat. Farmers also give livestock growth-producing hormones that include natural and synthetic versions of estrogen, progesterone, and testosterone, causing their weight to increase rapidly. This artificial plumping process boosts the amount of meat that farmers can sell per animal. Dairy cows are given the non-steroidal hormone bovine somatotropin (bST or rbST) to increase milk production.

We are hunters, and the meat we eat is mostly venison. Each fall, we fill our freezers with enough to last until next deer season. If we are going to purchase meat, it's primarily organic chicken. It's expensive, but we don't need to eat a lot of meat. We are not purists at all. We still enjoy Don's famous smoked barbeque ribs and brisket. After all, we are from Texas. The dairy products and eggs we purchase are organic. Many of the household cleaning products we use are free of toxins. I am still making small changes. Remember, the changes you make are your own choice. Do your research and make your own decisions. Read the label and look up those long words. You are building a healthy host - your body. It's hard for a foreign invader, whether internal or external, to create destruction in a healthy environment.

My goal is to create a healthy host - my body. Genes are segments of DNA that contain the code for a specific protein that functions in one or more types of cells in the body. They have information that determines everything from appearance to intelligence. You inherit genes from your parents. How a parent lives affects their children's genes. Not everything you inherit in your genes is permanent. The study of epigenetics shows us that we don't have to be doomed by our genes. You are what you eat. Let food be your medicine. Stress can activate adverse changes. Peace can undo the damage and create new, healthy neural pathways. Be active and awaken your best genes. Change your environment. Nature is a nurturer. Sunshine, walks in the woods, beautiful sunsets are free and create wholeness within. Your mind is at ease and free to dream. Love is the most potent, life-giving force in the universe. Love God with your whole heart. Love yourself as God loves you. Actively love others by giving them your time, undistracted attention, and kind words of affirmation. Be intentional about loving. Choose someone each day to bless with your best self. Creating health and happiness is not expensive. You are becoming healthy from the inside out.

Chapter 30

UNDERSTANDING DIVERSE AND COMPLEMENTARY OPTIONS

Conventional medicine or traditional medicine - According to the National Cancer Institute at the National Institute of Health, conventional medicine is a system in which medical doctors and other healthcare professionals treat symptoms and diseases using drugs, radiation, or surgery. www.cancer.gov

Alternative medicine - Treatments that are used instead of standard medical treatments. One example is using a special diet to treat cancer instead of anticancer drugs prescribed by an oncologist. www.cancer.gov

Complementary medicine - Treatments used along with standard medical treatments but are not considered standard treatments. One example is using acupuncture to help lessen some side-effects of cancer treatment. www.cancer.gov

Integrative Medicine or Integrative Health - brings conventional and complementary approaches together in a coordinated way. It emphasizes a holistic, patient-focused approach to health care and wellness - often including mental, emotional, functional, spiritual, social, and community aspects - and treat the whole person rather than, for example, one organ system. www.nccih.nih.gov

Listed here are a few resources I explored. By doing your own research, you will discover new, healthy options.

Breast Cancer Treatment Handbook, The Comprehensive Patient Navigation Guide, Judy C. Kneece, RN, OCN.
Understanding the disease, treatments, emotions, and recovery from breast cancer.

National Cancer Institute. www.cancer.gov 1-800-422-6237. A part of the National Institute of Health.

American Cancer Society. www.cancer.org 1-1800-227-2345. A cancer diagnosis can be scary – and overwhelming. Whether you need emotional support, the latest cancer information, a ride to chemo, or a place to stay when treatment is far away, they are here to help – 24 hours a day, seven days a week.

LIVESTRONG, www.livestrong.org The mission is to improve the lives of people affected by cancer now. They provide direct services and connect people with services they need.

National Comprehensive Cancer Network (NCCN), www.nccn.org/patients. Empowers you to make informed decisions at each step of your cancer journey.

Breast Cancer Conqueror - Health and Wellness Website. Hosted by Dr. Veronique Desaulniers, D. C. She has also authored a book, *Healing Breast Cancer Naturally: 7 Essential Steps to Beating Breast Cancer*. www.hopkinsmedicine.org Visit their health library. Search the topics that interest you.

The Truth About Cancer - thetruthaboutcancer.com A newsgroup devoted to presenting alternative or complementary treatment options. You will learn about a host of alternative or complementary medical treatments for cancer.

Dr. Josh Axe - www.draxe.com A chiropractic doctor, a certified doctor of natural medicine, and a clinical nutritionist with a passion for helping people eat healthily and live a healthy lifestyle.

Chris Wark - Author, speaker, and health coach. A resource for healing cancer with nutrition and natural therapies. www.chrisbeatcancer.com He wrote, *Chris Beat Cancer: A Comprehensive Plan for Healing Naturally*.

Pain, Perplexity, and Promotion, Bob Sorge. A prophetic interpretation of the Book of Job. You will find hope and affirmation in this book.

The Cancer-Fighting Kitchen, by Rebecca Katz, Second Edition. Nourishing, big flavor recipes for cancer treatment and recovery.

Dr. William LaValley, Austin, TX. www.lavalleymdprotocols.com Licensed by the Texas Medical Board (TMB) and the College of Physicians and Surgeons of Nova Scotia (CPSNS) from 1988 to present. He is a Functional Integrative Medicine physician, treating patients for over 28 years, and as a professional consultant to other physicians since the mid-1990s. Dr. LaValley develops advanced, evidence-based, molecularly-targeted treatment plans containing multiple protocol recommendations for physicians to receive, consider, and administer to their patients diagnosed with various types of cancers.

Memorial Sloan Kettering Cancer Center. www.mskcc.org Located in New York, New York. They care for people with all types of cancer, from the most common to the rarest. They offer integrative medicine therapies, classes, and workshops, including mind-body therapies, a group of healing techniques that enhance the mind's interactions with bodily function, induce relaxation, and improve overall health and well-being. Options include acupuncture, aromatherapy, massage therapy, meditation, music therapy, Qigong, Tai Chi, and Yoga. You may be able to locate integrative medicine classes like these in your area.

University of Texas MD Anderson Cancer Center. www.mdanderson.org Located in Houston, Texas. Devoted exclusively to cancer patient care, research, education, and prevention. They also offer integrative oncology physician consultations, acupuncture, exercise and physical activity consultations, health psychology, music therapy, nutrition consultations, and oncology massage.

Dr. Joseph Mercola, www.mercola.com. Alternative medicine proponent and osteopathic physician. Online natural health information articles and health newsletter.

The Whole-Food Guide for Breast Cancer Survivors - A Nutritional Approach to Prevent Recurrence, by Edward Bauman, Med, Ph.D. and Helayne Waldman, MS, EDD

Foods to Fight Cancer - Essential Foods to Prevent Cancer, by Richard Beliveau, Ph.D. and Denis Gingras, PhD.

Switch on Your Brain, A Key to Peak Happiness, Thinking, and Health, by Dr. Caroline Leaf. Your thinking affects your health.

Mindful Meditation: 30 Days Uniting with the Heart of God, by Jeanie Winebarger. Change your altitude. Don't stay stuck in the valley. Look up and climb that mountain. Your faith brings you fresh breezes of hope and health. You will be soaring with angel's wings, then reaching out to help others.

National Institute of Health U.S. National Library of Medicine at www.MedlinePlus.gov A free and open research-based resource.

National Institute of Health National Library of Medicine at www.PubMed.gov A free and open research-based resource.

Epilogue

The Poetic Warrior

When I was about ten years old, my teacher asked our fifth-grade class to choose a poem for memorization. I chose a poem by Henry Wadsworth Longfellow, an American poet who lived in the 1800s. I have never forgotten it. It is a poem about life and how to live it. The author sums up what it takes to live a successful life through tragedy and triumph!

A Psalm of Life
Tell me not, in mournful numbers,
Life is but an empty dream!
For the soul is dead that slumbers,
And things are not what they seem.

Life is real! Life is earnest!
And the grave is not its goal;
Dust thou art, to dust returnest,
Was not spoken of the soul.

Not enjoyment, and not sorrow,
Is our destined end or way;
But to act, that each tomorrow
Find us farther than today.

Art is long, and Time is fleeting,
And our hearts, though stout and brave,
Still, like muffled drums, are beating
Funeral marches to the grave.

In the world's broad field of battle,
In the bivouac of Life,
Be not like dumb, driven cattle!
Be a hero in the strife!

Trust no Future, howe'er pleasant!
Let the dead Past bury its dead!
Act,— act in the living Present!
Heart within, and God o'erhead!

Lives of great men all remind us
We can make our lives sublime,
And, departing, leave behind us
Footprints on the sands of time;

Footprints, that perhaps another,
Sailing o'er life's solemn main,
A forlorn and shipwrecked brother,
Seeing, shall take heart again.

Let us, then, be up and doing,
With a heart for any fate;
Still achieving, still pursuing,
Learn to labor and to wait.

Dear Reader, I bless you as you walk through the storms, the sunshine, the rain, the shadows, the darkness, the joys, the gladness, the sorrows, and the hope of each new day. Make yours a life well-lived. Pursue your purpose and passion. Make someone smile. Lift the weary. Live a life that really matters.

I see you now. Off you go, smiling and marching into your magnificent tomorrow!

Jean

www.ingramcontent.com/pod-product-compliance
Lightning Source LLC
Chambersburg PA
CBHW071504080526
44587CB00014B/2208